Second Edition

UNDERSTANDING LUNG SOUNDS

Steven Lehrer, M.D.

Staff Physician
Veterans Affairs Medical Center
Associate Professor, Mount Sinai School of Medicine
City University of New York
Bronx, New York

W. B. SAUNDERS COMPANY
A Division of Harcourt Brace & Company

Philadelphia/London/Toronto
Montreal/Sydney/Tokyo

W. B. SAUNDERS COMPANY
A Division of
Harcourt Brace & Company

The Curtis Center
Independence Square West
Philadelphia, PA 19106

Library of Congress Cataloging-in-Publication Data

Lehrer, Steven.
  Understanding lung sounds / Steven Lehrer. — 2nd ed.
    p. cm.
  Includes bibliographical references and index.

  ISBN 0-7216-4902-5

  1. Auscultation. 2. Lungs—Sounds. 3. Lungs—
Examination.
  I. Title. [DNLM: 1. Auscultation. 2. Respiratory
  Sounds—diagnosis. WF 141 L524u 1993]
RC734.A94L43 1993   616.2′407544—dc20
DNLM/DLC   92-48450

Cover Illustration by Edward M. Jones

Understanding Lung Sounds   ISBN 0-7216-4902-5

Printed in the United States of America

Last digit is the print
number: 9   8   7   6   5   4   3   2   1

FOREWORD

Physicians have been listening to lung sounds since several centuries before Christ; witness the succussion splash of hydropneumothorax, which is attributed to Hippocrates. In 1816, Laennec's substitution of the stethoscope for direct application of the ear to the chest ushered in a Golden Age. The phenomenology of abnormal lung sounds was brought to bear on the diagnosis of lung cavities, consolidation, emphysema, and pleural effusions. The Golden Age lasted out the century. Although the importance of stethoscopy in the clinical armamentarium continues to this day, as indicated in this book, the method was partially eclipsed by the advent of the x-ray in 1895, followed by the derivative methods of pulmonary arteriography in the 1950s and CT scanning in the 1970s. Indeed, the eclipse has probably gone too far, for the availability and ease of use of the stethoscope are hard to beat. Thus, Dr. Lehrer's book is an important one.

In parallel with the description of the phenomena of lung sounds has been the science of lung sounds. Correlations with the findings of autopsy (Laennec himself initiated this approach) and later correlations with the radiographic findings constituted the main basis of that science, but some studies of the physics of lung sounds date back into the last century. More recent physical studies include the analyses I made by the method of sound spectrography in the 1950s. The physics of lung sounds continues to absorb the interest of a small but avid group of clinical scientists. Indeed, the 8th International Conference on Lung Sounds was held here at Johns Hopkins in September, 1983, assembling aficionados from many countries to review their work in this field.

It is the art and science of lung sounds that Steve Lehrer brings together in this useful book on a persistently important part of our clinical armamentarium.

VICTOR A. McKUSICK, M.D.
William Osler Professor and Director,
Department of Medicine,
Johns Hopkins University
    School of Medicine;
Physician-in-Chief,
Johns Hopkins Hospital, Baltimore, Md.

PREFACE

Since antiquity, physicians have examined the chest for signs of disease. Some physical diagnostic signs that are recognized today were first noted by the ancient Greeks. In the 18th century, percussion techniques were added to the diagnostic repertoire, and in the 19th century, auscultation was added. For many years, these methods, along with a carefully elicited history, were the only tools available to diagnose chest diseases.

The situation changed dramatically in 1895 with the discovery of x-rays. Suddenly, many chest structures could be observed, as through a window. Diagnosis became considerably more refined and simple to accomplish; all one needed to do was to inspect the x-ray film. The teaching of physical diagnosis of the chest, especially auscultation and the recognition of normal and abnormal breath sounds, received little attention except from chest specialists.

In the past few years, however, interest in breath sounds has been growing. Breath sound analytic techniques, drawing on modern electronic and acoustic advances, have become increasingly sophisticated. Some researchers hope eventually to construct a computerized electronic device able to "listen" to the chest and then produce a data printout of information that can now be obtained only with multiple pulmonary function tests.

The purpose of this book is to teach elementary chest diagnosis and, above all, how to listen to breath sounds. Much new information on the significance of normal and abnormal breath sounds can be found here. In addition, the latest research findings are presented, along with the most significant data, often in graphic form, from each investigator's work. To help the beginning student, some concepts from anatomy, physiology, and pathology are presented; however, this material is not intended to be a complete treatise on the lung. It is only meant to provide enough background information to elucidate the remaining material. Full, detailed discussions of anatomy, physiology, and pathology may be found in the works listed in the bibliography for Chapter 1.

I am grateful to many individuals for the help they gave me while I was writing this book. Dr. David W. Cugell, Dr. Earle B. Weiss, the American College of Chest Physicians, Dr. A. R. Nath, Dr. Steve S. Kraman, Dr. Peter Krumpe, Dr. Roy Donnerberg, Dr. Rand David, and Dr. Marilyn Orenstein provided sounds for the tape accompanying this volume. Gary Hilt helped with the recording of sounds. Margaret Kinney, Kathleen O'Hogan, and Loyola Salva, of the Bronx VA Hospital Medical Library, found many articles for me. Katherine Pitcoff, Frances T. Mues, Anna Congdon, and Betty Gittens, all formerly of the W. B. Saunders Company provided much invaluable editorial guidance. Dr. David W. Cugell, Dr. Steve S. Kraman, and Dr. Marvin Lesser reviewed the entire manuscript and made many helpful suggestions. Edward M. Jones prepared the original illustrations. Gloria Spevacek, of the Bronx VA Hospital Medical Media Production Service, obtained some of the reference material for me. Blandine Triestman of W. B. Saunders Company was a constant source of support and encouragement.

A final word is in order about the title of this book. The sounds of breathing may be described by three synonymous terms: *lung sounds, breath sounds,* and *respiratory sounds. Lung sounds* is the term often used by researchers. *Breath sounds* is the term frequently employed by physicians, nurses, and respiratory therapists involved in direct patient care. *Respiratory sounds* is the index term used for classification in the *Index Medicus,* which lists all articles on the subject under this one heading. In the following chapters, the three terms will be used interchangeably.

STEVEN LEHRER

PREFACE TO THE SECOND EDITION

Numerous advances in the study of lung sounds have occurred since the first edition of *Understanding Lung Sounds* was published. There has been progress in lung sound analysis with the advent of a computer method, fast Fourier transformation. At least one new diagnostic sign has been described: poor breath sounds with good voice sounds in bronchial stenosis. And investigators have done comparative analyses of adult and infant lung sounds, noting especially the frequency differences. These and other areas of research are described in this second edition.

I thank Dr. Steve S. Kraman and Pamela Dunn Lehrer for their help in the preparation of this revision. I am also grateful to Mr. Thomas Eoyang, of W. B. Saunders Company, for his suggestions and support.

STEVEN LEHRER, M.D.
New York City
December 1992

CONTENTS

1

THE LUNGS

Anatomy, Physiology, and Pathology Relevant to Breath Sounds

The purpose of the lung is gas exchange. Its most important function is to allow oxygen to move from the air into the systemic venous blood to meet the metabolic needs of the cells; the lung then allows carbon dioxide, a waste product of cellular metabolism, to move out. This function is accomplished through a series of complex processes. Contraction of the inspiratory muscles results in flow of air through the trachea and bronchi into the alveoli of the lung. Here, alveolar air and pulmonary capillary blood, though separated by an ultrathin alveolar–capillary membrane, come into very close contact. Oxygen diffuses across the alveolar–capillary membrane into the blood while carbon dioxide passes in the opposite direction.

ANATOMY

The lungs are cone-shaped organs that completely fill the pleural spaces. The right lung is divided by fissures into an upper, a middle, and a lower lobe. The left lung is divided into an upper and a lower lobe. Air moves into and out of the lungs through the airways, which are subdivided into two components from a functional point of view: (1) the conducting airways, often called the tracheobronchial tree, consisting of the trachea, the bronchi, and the bronchioles; and (2) the terminal respiratory units (sometimes called the acini; Fig. 1–1). The conducting airways function chiefly to conduct gas into and out of the terminal respiratory units, where the actual gas exchange takes place.

1

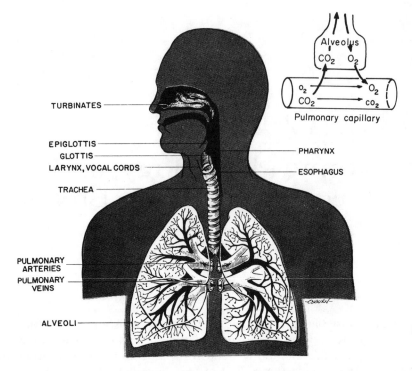

TURBINATES

EPIGLOTTIS
GLOTTIS
LARYNX, VOCAL CORDS

TRACHEA

PULMONARY
ARTERIES
PULMONARY
VEINS

ALVEOLI

Alveolus
CO_2 O_2

O_2
CO_2 O_2
CO_2

Pulmonary capillary

PHARYNX

ESOPHAGUS

FIGURE 1–1.   The respiratory passages.   (From Guyton AC: *Textbook of Medical Physiology*. 8th ed. Philadelphia, WB Saunders Company, 1991, p 410.)

CONDUCTING AIRWAYS

Air enters the gas-exchanging units of the lung by way of the nose or mouth, then passes through the larynx and tracheobronchial system. The upper air passages filter, humidify, and adjust the temperature of inspired air.

TRACHEA

The extrathoracic portion of the trachea lies in the midline of the anterior part of the neck. After entering the thorax, the trachea deviates slightly to the right. The trachea is supported by horseshoe-shaped rings of cartilage, connected posteriorly by a pliable membrane. During coughing, the increased pressure within the thorax pushes the membrane into the space between the arms of the cartilages, narrowing the lumen significantly. Consequently, velocity of air flow increases, creating a shearing force that dislodges material lying on the mucosal surface.

The trachea divides into the right and left main bronchi at the carina. The right bronchus leaves the bifurcation at less of an angle than does the left bronchus; for this reason, aspirated fluids are more prone to enter the right lung. As the right-sided displacement of the trachea within the thorax carries it away from the left lung and closer to the right, the left main bronchus is longer (5 cm) than the right (3 cm).

The bronchi are divided into lobar and segmental branches (Fig. 1–2). Familiarity with these divisions, especially the bronchopulmonary segments, is important, because some lung diseases are characteristically found within particular segments. For example, pulmonary tuberculosis is most likely to affect the apical and posterior upper lobe segments or the superior segment of the lower lobes.

A bronchopulmonary segment is a wedge of lung tissue that is supplied by a single segmental bronchus and its corresponding pulmonary artery. The venous drainage of the segments is variable, with a vein often draining more than one segment. Each segment functions as a relatively independent unit, although there is some collateral circulation and ventilation between adjacent segments. The segments are irregular in shape and variable in size and are separated by thin, incomplete connective tissue barriers.

The bronchi subdivide into smaller and smaller passages, referred to as generations. The last and smallest branches, from which the terminal respiratory units originate, are called terminal bronchioles. Near the hilum of the lung, the terminal bronchioles may be reached with only 10 bronchial branchings; more than 25 branchings may be necessary to reach the terminal bronchioles in the most peripheral basal parts of the lung.

TERMINAL RESPIRATORY UNITS

The terminal bronchioles are joined to the terminal respiratory units, also known as the lung parenchyma; here, gas exchange takes place. A group of three to five terminal bronchioles, each with its appended terminal respiratory unit, is usually called a pulmonary lobule.

Terminal respiratory units, sometimes called acini or primary lobules, have a characteristically variable branching pattern. There are usually two to five orders of respiratory bronchioles, the last of which leads to two to five orders of alveolar ducts. Each alveolar duct leads to 10 to 16 alveoli (Fig. 1–3). An average adult has 300 million alveoli, but this figure is highly variable, depending on age and body size. Because 90% of the total alveolar surface is covered with pulmonary capillaries, the alveolar capillary surface available for gas exchange is 60 to 70

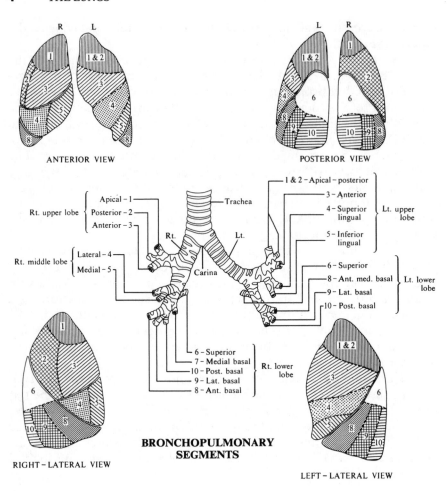

ANTERIOR VIEW

POSTERIOR VIEW

Rt. upper lobe { Apical – 1
Posterior – 2
Anterior – 3

Trachea

1 & 2 – Apical – posterior
3 – Anterior
4 – Superior lingual
5 – Inferior lingual } Lt. upper lobe

Rt.

Lt.

Rt. middle lobe { Lateral – 4
Medial – 5

Carina

6 – Superior
8 – Ant. med. basal
9 – Lat. basal
10 – Post. basal } Lt. lower lobe

6 – Superior
7 – Medial basal
10 – Post. basal
9 – Lat. basal
8 – Ant. basal } Rt. lower lobe

**BRONCHOPULMONARY
SEGMENTS**

RIGHT – LATERAL VIEW

LEFT – LATERAL VIEW

RIGHT – MEDIAL VIEW

LEFT – MEDIAL VIEW

FIGURE 1–2. The trachea and the bronchopulmonary segments. (From Pansky B, House EL: *Review of Gross Anatomy.* 3rd ed. New York, Macmillan Publishing Company, 1975, p 279.)

FIGURE 1–3.   Structure of the lung. A, anatomic alveolus; AD, alveolar duct; RB, respiratory bronchiole; TB, terminal bronchiole.   (From Staub NC: The pathophysiology of pulmonary edema. *Hum Pathol* *1:*419, 1970.)

square meters in the normal adult (1 square meter per kilogram of body weight).

   Gas in the alveoli does not contact the alveolar epithelium directly; instead, the surface is covered by a layer of fluid containing a substance called surfactant, which imparts the lowest surface tension of any biologic material ever tested. Low surface tension at this location is important; it keeps alveoli from collapsing. When surfactant is deficient, as in the neonatal respiratory distress syndrome, atelectasis and severe mechanical disturbances occur. Surfactant is a phospholipid that is secreted by special cells of the alveolar epithelium.

CHEST WALL

The thorax, that part of the body between the neck and abdomen, is encased by a bony framework of ribs shaped like a truncated cone and lined by the pleura, a fibrous membrane. Between the ribs lie two bands of muscles, the external and internal intercostals. The external intercostal muscles extend from the articulations between the ribs and vertebral bodies to the origins of the costal cartilages. The internal intercostals extend from the sternum to the angles of the ribs. Normal inspiratory breathing at rest is performed by contraction of the muscles of inspiration—the diaphragm and external intercostals; normal expiration is passive and requires no muscular effort. However, when increased amounts of air are necessary, expiration in normal people becomes active; accessory muscles of respiration in the neck—sternocleidomastoids and scalene—as well as abdominal muscles—rectus, external and internal obliques, and transversus abdominis—are utilized to augment the rate and depth of breathing. Patients with certain lung diseases, such as asthma and emphysema, often need to use expiratory muscles and accessory muscles to maintain adequate ventilation at rest.

PHYSIOLOGY

The process of respiration can be divided into three major mechanistic events: (1) pulmonary ventilation—the inflow and outflow of air between the atmosphere and lung alveoli; (2) diffusion of oxygen and carbon dioxide between the alveoli and the blood; and (3) transport of oxygen and carbon dioxide in the blood and body fluids to and from the cells. Only those aspects of pulmonary ventilation that are most pertinent to an understanding of breath sounds will be discussed here.

During inspiration at rest, the intra-alveolar pressure becomes slightly negative with respect to atmospheric pressure, normally slightly less than -1 mm Hg, and this causes air to flow inward through the respiratory passageways. During normal expiration at rest, the intra-alveolar pressure rises to slightly less than $+1$ mm Hg, causing air to flow outward through the respiratory passageways.

The lungs have a continual elastic tendency to collapse and recoil away from the chest wall. Two different factors cause this tendency: (1) elastic fibers throughout the lung that are stretched during inflation, and (2) surface tension of the fluid lining the alveoli, which tends to pull them closed. Without the presence of the previously mentioned surfactant to reduce this surface tension, lung expansion would be extremely difficult.

The compliance of the lungs and thorax is expressed as the volume increase in the lungs for each unit increase in transpulmonary pressure. The compliance of the normal lungs and thorax combined is 0.08 to 0.10 liter per cm of water pressure. In other words, when the alveolar pressure is increased by 1 cm water, the lungs expand 80 to 100 ml.

The lungs alone, when removed from the chest, are almost twice as distensible as the lungs and thorax together, because the thoracic cage must also be stretched when the lungs are expanded within it. Thus, the muscles of inspiration use energy both to expand the lungs and to expand the thoracic cage around the lungs. Many pathologic conditions affecting the lung cause decreased compliance. These include deformities of the thoracic cage, such as kyphosis or scoliosis, fibrosis, and interstitial fibrosis.

As has been mentioned, during ordinary quiet breathing, muscle contraction occurs only during inspiration; expiration is entirely passive, resulting from elastic recoil of the lung and thorax. The work of inspiration can be divided into two fractions: (1) compliance work, necessary to expand the lung against its elastic forces; and (2) airway and tissue resistance work, needed to overcome the viscosity of lung, chest wall structures, and airway resistance during movement of air into the lungs. These two types of work are illustrated graphically in Figure 1–4. As can be seen, during normal quiet breathing, most of the work done by the respiratory muscles is done merely to expand the lungs (compliance work). But during very heavy breathing, when air must flow through the airways at high velocity, the greatest proportion of the work goes to overcome airway resistance. During normal quiet breathing, only 2% to 3% of the total body energy requirement, measured by oxygen consumption, is needed for pulmonary ventilation; but in the presence of some severe pulmonary diseases such as asthma and emphysema, a third or more of total body energy must be expended for the same purpose.

A simple technique for recording the volume movement of air into and out of the lungs is called *spirometry*. A typical spirometer consists of a drum inverted over a chamber of water, with the drum counterbalanced by a weight (Fig. 1–5). The drum contains a breathing mixture of gases, usually air or oxygen; the mouth is connected to the gas chamber by a tube. When the subject breathes in and out of the cham-

FIGURE 1–4. Graphic representation of the two different types of work accomplished during inspiration: (1) compliance work, the largest fraction, represented by the trapezoid OAECDO and (2) airway and tissue resistance work, represented by the hatched area ABCEA. (From West JB: *Respiratory Physiology—The Essentials.* 2nd ed. Baltimore, Williams & Wilkins, 1979, p 112.)

FIGURE 1-5. A spirometer. (From Guyton AC: *Textbook of Medical Physiology.* 8th ed. Philadelphia, WB Saunders Company, 1991, p 407.)

ber, the drum rises and falls, and a recording is made on a moving sheet of paper.

Figure 1-6 is a diagram demonstrating changes in lung volume under different conditions of breathing. In this diagram, air in the lungs has been subdivided into four different volumes and four different capacities (predicted values depend on age, sex, and height).

FIGURE 1-6. Diagram showing respiratory excursions during normal breathing and during maximal inspiration and maximal expiration. (From Guyton AC: *Textbook of Medical Physiology.* 8th ed. Philadelphia, WB Saunders Company, 1991, p 407.)

1. The tidal volume = volume of air inspired or expired with each normal breath, usually about 500 ml.
2. The inspiratory reserve volume = extra volume of air that can be inspired over and beyond the normal tidal volume, usually about 3000 ml.
3. The expiratory reserve volume = amount of air that can still be expired by forceful expiration after the end of a normal tidal expiration, usually about 1100 ml.
4. The residual volume = volume of air still remaining in the lungs after the most forceful expiration, usually about 1200 ml.

When these four volumes are added together, they are equal to the maximum volume to which the lungs can be expanded. When two or more of the aforementioned volumes are considered together, they are called pulmonary capacities.

1. The inspiratory capacity = tidal volume + inspiratory reserve volume, about 3500 ml. This is the amount of air that a subject can breathe beginning at the normal expiratory level and distending the lungs maximally.
2. The functional residual capacity = expiratory reserve volume + residual volume, about 2300 ml. This is the amount of air remaining in the lungs at the end of normal expiration.
3. The vital capacity = inspiratory reserve volume + tidal volume + expiratory reserve volume, about 4600 ml. This is the maximum amount of air that a subject can expel from the lungs after they are first filled to the maximum extent and then expired to the maximum extent.
4. The total lung capacity = the maximum volume to which the lungs can be expanded with the greatest possible inspiratory effort, about 5800 ml (this includes vital capacity and residual volume).

When all inspiratory muscles are completely relaxed, the lungs return to a resting state called the resting expiratory level. The volume of air in the lungs is then equal to the functional residual capacity, about 2300 ml in the young adult.

Each of the pulmonary volumes and capacities has a specific significance. Moreover, each changes with the position of the body; most decrease when the subject lies down and increase when the subject stands up. Two factors account for this change: (1) the abdominal contents press upward against the diaphragm in the lying position, and (2) pulmonary blood volume increases in the lying position. Both of these changes decrease the space available for pulmonary air.

The residual volume, the air that cannot be removed from the lungs even by forceful expiration, furnishes air in the alveoli to aerate the blood, even between breaths. Were there no residual volume, the concentrations of oxygen and carbon dioxide in the blood would rise and fall markedly with each breath.

Any of the following abnormalities tends to diminish the vital capacity:

1. *Paralysis of the respiratory muscles.* This often occurs after spinal cord injuries or poliomyelitis and can decrease vital capacity to 1000 to 500 ml.
2. *Diminished pulmonary compliance ("stiff lungs").* Tuberculosis, lung cancer, and pulmonary fibrosis can all reduce pulmonary compliance and thereby decrease vital capacity.
3. *Pulmonary vascular congestion.* In left heart failure or any other condition causing pulmonary vascular congestion and edema, vital capacity is reduced because excess fluid in the lungs decreases compliance.

Another very important measurement of ventilatory function is the *maximum expiratory flow rate*. When a person expires with progressively increasing force, the expiratory air flow rate reaches a maximum, despite still further increase in expiratory force. This effect can be understood by referring to Figure 1–7A. When pressure is applied to the lungs by chest cage compression, the same amount of pressure is applied to the exterior of both the alveoli and the respiratory passages, as indicated by the arrows. Consequently, not only is the pressure increased in the alveoli to force air to the exterior, but the terminal bronchioles are collapsed at the same time, increasing airway resistance. Beyond a certain point, these two effects have equal but opposite results on air flow.

Figure 1–7B illustrates this phenomenon. The plotted curve is the expiratory flow achieved by a normal subject who first inhales as much air as possible and then expires with maximum effort until he can expire no further. Note that an expiratory air flow of over 400 liters per minute is rapidly reached. However, no matter how much further effort is exerted, this is the maximum expiratory flow that can be achieved.

Note also that as lung volume decreases, maximum expiratory flow decreases, principally because in the enlarged lung, the bronchi are held open partially by elastic pull on their exteriors by structural elements of the lung. However, as the lung becomes smaller, these structures are relaxed, and the bronchi collapse more easily.

Maximum expiratory flow-volume curves are often recorded in the pulmonary function laboratory to determine ventilatory abnormalities. In restrictive disease (constricted lungs), both total lung capacity (TLC) and residual volume (RV) are diminished. In addition,

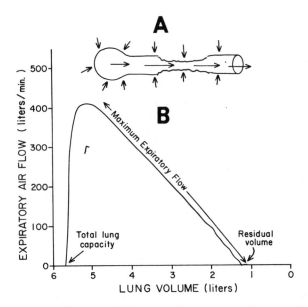

FIGURE 1–7.   (*A*) Collapse of the respiratory passageway during maximal expiratory effort; this effect limits the expiratory flow rate. (*B*) Effect of lung volume on the maximal expiratory air flow; note the decreasing maximal expiratory air flow as the lung volume becomes smaller.   (From Guyton AC: *Textbook of Medical Physiology*. 8th ed. Philadelphia, WB Saunders Company, 1991, p 455.)

as the lung cannot expand to its normal volume, even with the greatest expiratory effort, the maximal expiratory flow rate cannot rise to normal. Among the restrictive lung diseases are advanced tuberculosis and silicosis; also included are diffuse interstitial pulmonary fibrosis of unknown etiology; kyphosis and scoliosis, which constrict the chest cage; drug-induced fibrotic reactions; and fibrosis secondary to chemical or physical injury.

In the presence of airway obstruction, expiration is usually much more difficult than inspiration because the expiratory closing tendency of the airways is greatly increased, whereas the negative intrapleural pressure of inspiration actually "pulls" the airways open. Consequently, air tends to enter the lung easily, where it becomes trapped. Moreover, because many airways are partially obstructed and because they collapse more easily than normal airways, maximum expiratory flow is markedly diminished. Severe airway obstruction occurs in asthma, chronic bronchitis, bronchiectasis, and emphysema.

A simple, useful test of airway obstruction is the *forced expiratory vital capacity* (FVC). Recordings of FVC, made on a spirometer, are shown in Figure 1–8A for a subject with normal lungs, and in Figure 1–8B for a subject with respiratory obstruction. To obtain the recording, the examiner asks the subject to inspire maximally to total lung capacity, then to exhale into the spirometer with maximum expiratory effort as rapidly and completely as possible. The total excursion of the record represents the forced vital capacity, as illustrated in the figure.

In normal lungs and lungs with obstructed airways, the forced vital capacities may be equal, but often they are not, owing in part to air trapping. In addition, there is a marked difference in the flow rate at which the subjects can expire, especially within the first second. This forced expiratory volume during the first second (FEV1) is recorded and used for comparison between normal and abnormal. In a normal subject, the forced vital capacity expired in the first second (FEV1/FVC %) is about 80%. However, in the subject with airway obstruction shown in Figure 1–8B, this value has decreased to only 47%. In severe airway obstruction, often seen in acute asthma, the value can decrease to less than 20%.

The most important factor in the entire ventilatory process is the rate at which the air is renewed each minute by atmospheric air in the gas-exchange area of the lungs—the alveoli, the alveolar sacs, the alveolar ducts, and the respiratory bronchioles; this process is called alveolar ventilation. Obviously, considerably less gas flows into the alveoli than flows into the lungs, because a large portion of the inspired air goes to fill respiratory passageways, the membranes of which are not

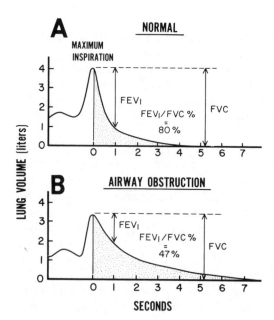

FIGURE 1–8. Spirometer recordings made during a forced vital capacity test in a normal subject (*A*), and in a subject with airway obstruction (*B*). (From Guyton AC: *Textbook of Medical Physiology.* 8th ed. Philadelphia, WB Saunders Company, 1991, p 456.)

capable of significant gaseous exchange with the blood. This air is referred to as dead-space air. No breath sounds are believed to be produced by alveolar ventilation.

The mechanisms that produce abnormal breath sounds may be best comprehended with an understanding of the major pathologic processes and alterations that can occur in the lung. A brief description of these is presented here.

ATELECTASIS. Atelectasis is a condition in which a portion of the lungs is unexpanded. A whole lung, a lobe, or only small segments within a lobe may be involved. Congenital atelectasis is failure of the lungs to expand fully in the neonatal period. Functional atelectasis results from incomplete inflation of the lungs during quiet breathing.

Acquired atelectasis is either obstructive or compressive. Obstructive atelectasis results from an obstruction of the trachea or bronchi; it may be caused by aspiration of a foreign body, a tumor mass occluding the bronchus, or exudate. A large area of atelectasis, often called massive collapse, may cause the heart to be displaced to the affected side. Compressive atelectasis results from compression of the lung by fluid or air in the pleural or pericardial space, a large intrathoracic tumor (Fig. 1–9), or elevation of the diaphragm. When the ate-

FIGURE 1–9. Atelectasis of the left upper lobe. Posteroanterior (A) and lateral (B) views of left upper lobe atelectasis (arrows) from squamous cell carcinoma. The triangular shadow with concave borders on the lateral view is characteristic. (From Hinshaw HC, Murray JF: *Diseases of the Chest.* 4th ed. Philadelphia, WB Saunders Company, 1980, p 616.)

lectatic lung expands, crackles are heard through the stethoscope because of the sudden opening of airways (see Chapter 5).

EMPHYSEMA.   Emphysema is an abnormal enlargement of the air spaces accompanied by destruction of the alveolar walls; these changes produce considerable increase in the volume of the lungs (Fig. 1–10). Emphysema usually requires many years to develop into the advanced stages characterized by shortness of breath and barrel chest. The physical findings include increase in anteroposterior diameter of the chest, fixation of the chest with the ribs in a more nearly horizontal plane, and use of the accessory muscles of respiration. Diminished breath sounds are heard through the stethoscope (see Chapter 5). In the Western world, cigarette smoking is virtually the only cause of emphysema. The single significant exception is alpha-l-antitrypsin deficiency, an enzyme deficiency, which is rare.

CONSOLIDATION.   Consolidation, which is a solidifying of lung tissue because of the presence of large amounts of fluid, is a hallmark of pneumonia. Bronchial breath sounds, egophony, whispered pectoriloquy, and bronchophony are heard over a consolidated lung (Fig. 1–11; see Chapter 5).

FIGURE 1–10.   Roentgenographic findings in emphysema. (A) Posteroanterior and (B) lateral chest x-rays of a 62-year-old woman with advanced chronic obstructive pulmonary disease, mainly emphysema, showing low flattened diaphragms, large retrosternal air space, vertically oriented heart, and hyperlucent lung fields.   (From Hinshaw HC, Murray JF: *Diseases of the Chest*. 4th ed. Philadelphia, WB Saunders Company, 1980, p 578.)

FIGURE 1-11.   Consolidation in three cases of verified pneumococcal pneumonia involving the right upper lobe (*A* and *B*), the right middle lobe (*C* and *D*), and the right lower lobe (*E* and *F*).   (From Hinshaw HC, Murray JF: *Diseases of the Chest.* 4th ed. Philadelphia, WB Saunders Company, 1980, p 254.)

PNEUMOTHORAX.   Pneumothorax occurs when air enters the pleural space, permitting partial or total collapse of a lung, often in otherwise normal young people. Air escapes into the pleural cavity because of rupture of a distended bleb on the surface of the lung. Pneumothorax may also result from laceration of the lung due to a fractured rib, a puncture wound, or tuberculosis (Fig. 1–12). Breath sounds will be absent over one side of the chest when a lung is totally collapsed. Patients with pneumothorax generally note the rapid onset of pleuritic type chest pain associated with some difficulty in breathing. There is hyperresonance to percussion on the side of lung collapse (see Chapter 3), and the trachea may deviate toward the opposite side of the chest.

PLEURAL FLUID.   Fluid in the pleural cavity can accumulate as the result of excessive production, interference with the drainage mechanisms that normally keep the pleural space relatively dry, or a combination of both (Fig. 1–13). Inflammatory processes, alteration in venous or lymphatic flow, or changes in serum oncotic pressure can produce fluid accumulation between the pleural surfaces. Any substantial accumulation of fluid between these surfaces interferes with the transmission of breath sounds and vocal sounds; it also impairs resonance. When there is sufficient fluid accumulation to produce some compression of the underlying lung, the breath sound characteristics are altered (see Chapter 5). Breath sounds will be absent over a large effusion.

FIGURE 1–12.   Small pneumothorax. Detailed views of right upper lung and chest wall. Note that the air gap (arrows) is wider and more apparent in expiration (*A*) than in inspiration (*B*). (From Hinshaw HC, Murray JF: *Diseases of the Chest.* 4th ed. Philadelphia, WB Saunders Company, 1980, p 905.)

FIGURE 1–13.   (*A*) X-ray demonstrating massive pleural effusion in right hemithorax in a cancer patient with pleural metastases. (*B*) Film made one month after treatment. Patient's pleural effusion is diminished and shortness of breath relieved.   (From Camishion RC, Gibbon JH, Nealon TF: Talc poudrage in the treatment of pleural effusion due to cancer. *Surg Clin North Am* 42:1521, 1962.)

STUDY HELPS

1. Why are aspirated fluids and inhaled foreign bodies more prone to enter the right lung?
2. What is the function of surfactant? What disease occurs when it is deficient?
3. During ordinary quiet breathing, why is muscle activity needed only for inspiration?
4. Describe a spirometer. What is its function?
5. What diseases commonly produce restricted pulmonary function?
6. What pulmonary function tests are used for estimating the degree of respiratory obstruction?
7. Which abnormalities tend to diminish the vital capacity?

BIBLIOGRAPHY

BATES DV, MACKLEM PT, CHRISTIE RV: *Respiratory Function in Disease*. Philadelphia, WB Saunders Company, 1971.

COMROE JH: *The Lung: Clinical Physiology and Pulmonary Function Tests*. 2nd ed. Chicago, Year Book Medical Publishers, 1962.

COMROE JH: *Physiology of Respiration*. 2nd ed. Chicago, Year Book Medical Publishers, 1962.

DIVERTIE MB, BRASS A (ed): *Respiratory System*. Summit, NJ, Ciba, 1979.

GUYTON AC: *Textbook of Medical Physiology*. 8th ed. Philadelphia, WB Saunders Company, 1991.

HINSHAW HC, MURRAY JF: *Diseases of the Chest*. 4th ed. Philadelphia, WB Saunders Company, 1980.

PRIOR JA, Silberstein JS: *Physical Diagnosis*. 6th ed. St Louis, CV Mosby Company, 1981.

WEST JB: *Respiratory Physiology—The Essentials*. 2nd ed. Baltimore, Williams & Wilkins, 1979.

2

SOUND, HEARING, AND THE STETHOSCOPE

The Nature of Sound

Sounds consist of audible vibrations created by alternating regions of compression and rarefaction of air. To see what a sound wave looks like, one may mount a pen on one prong of a vibrating tuning fork and then run a piece of paper under the pen. The pen will inscribe an S-shaped wave called a sine wave. The peaks and valleys in the wave correspond to the alternating regions of compression and rarefaction that make up the sound wave (Fig. 2–1). Sound has three principal characteristics: frequency, intensity, and duration (Fig. 2–2).

Frequency is a measure of the number of vibrations per unit time, in cycles per second or hertz (Hz). A large number of vibrations, as in a high-frequency wheeze, will yield a sound that is subjectively interpreted by the examiner as being high-pitched. A low-frequency wheeze, on the other hand, will give a sound that is heard as low-pitched.

Intensity is governed by four factors: (1) the amplitude of the vibrations, (2) the source producing the energy, (3) the distance the vibrations must travel, and (4) the medium through which they travel. These factors determine whether a sound is perceived as loud or faint. For example, breath sounds are much fainter than normal over an emphysematous lung, because the damaged, hyperaerated tissue conducts sound poorly.

Duration of the vibrations determines whether the ear interprets them as short or long, for example, a short wheeze or a long wheeze.

A fourth characteristic, *quality*, also known as timbre, is a result of the component frequencies that make up any particular sound. Quality allows one to perceive the difference in the same note played on a violin or on a piano (Fig. 2–3). In the chest, quality allows the examiner to distinguish between a vesicular and a bronchial breath sound (see

19

FIGURE 2–1. The vibrating tuning fork produces the sound wave shown (top), which consists of alternating areas of compressed and rarefied air. The changing pressure in these areas corresponds to the sine wave below. (From Rushmer RF: *Cardiac Diagnosis: A Physiologic Approach*. Philadelphia, WB Saunders Company, 1955, p 209.)

FIGURE 2–2.   (*A*) The frequency of vibration is determined by the relationship between mass and elasticity of the vibrating body; as shown in the example here, the larger mass (upper drawing) vibrates at a lower frequency. (*B*) The amplitude of the vibration and the corresponding intensity of the sound depend on the amount of displacement of the vibrating body; a high-intensity sound is produced by a large displacement (upper drawing). (*C*) The quality or timbre of the sound is a result of the relative intensity of the component frequencies that make up the vibration. Shown here is a high-frequency sine wave (overtone) superimposed on a low-frequency sine wave (the fundamental). (*D*) The duration of a vibration after the source of energy is cut off is dependent on the level of the energy and the rate at which it is dissipated. Note that each peak in the sine wave, going from left to right, is lower than the one before, indicating that the sound is diminishing progressively in amplitude. (From Rushmer RF: *Cardiac Diagnosis: A Physiologic Approach*. Philadelphia, WB Saunders Company, 1955, p 210.)

FIGURE 2-3. Wave form and sound spectrum for two stringed instruments—the violin and the piano. The fundamental frequency for both is 440 Hz (concert A). Four cycles of each wave are shown. The sound spectrum beneath each wave demonstrates the harmonic components of the wave. Note the presence of loud higher harmonics, especially the fifth, in the violin spectrum. (Reprinted by permission of Halliday D, Resnick R: *Physics*. New York, John Wiley & Sons, 1966.)

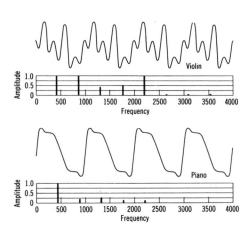

Chapters 4 and 5). E to A egophony (see Chapter 5) occurs because the quality of the voice sound heard through the stethoscope depends on whether the sound is being transmitted through normal or consolidated lung tissue.

Musical notes and breath sounds are made up of several frequency components. In a musical note, each of these components, which are simple multiples of one another, is called a harmonic; in most breath sounds, the relationship of the components is more complex, although a wheeze is quite analogous to a musical note. The pitch of a sound is determined by the component of lowest frequency, called the fundamental. The quality of a sound is determined by the higher frequency components, called overtones in a musical sound (Fig. 2-4).

In music, frequency or pitch is often expressed in terms of octaves above or below a given pitch, such as middle C. In the case of breath sounds, however, the number of cycles per second (Hz) is the preferred unit. The frequency range of the piano keyboard and its relationship to the range of breath sounds are shown in Figure 2-5.

FIGURE 2-4. A vibrating string, fixed at both ends, showing the first four modes of vibration. The uppermost mode produces the fundamental tone; the lower three modes generate the overtones. (Reprinted by permission of Halliday D, Resnick R: *Physics*. New York, John Wiley & Sons, 1966.)

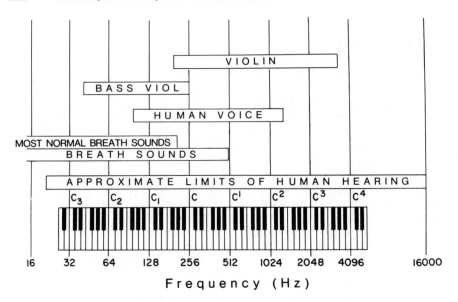

FIGURE 2-5.   The frequency range of the piano keyboard and its relationship to the range of breath sounds. Note that most breath sounds fall into the region below 200 Hz.   (Adapted from Butterworth JS, et al: Cardiac Auscultation Including Audio-visual Principles. New York, Grune & Stratton, 1955. Used by permission.)

HEARING

Most breath sounds fall into a frequency range to which the ear is relatively insensitive. Some of the basic physiology of hearing will be presented to clarify this point.

The eardrum is mechanically coupled to the cochlear apparatus by the three tiny bones (malleus, incus, and stapes) of the middle ear, called the ossicles (Fig. 2–6). The cochlea is essentially a selective sound frequency transducer, and a remarkably sensitive one. The eardrum need move only a distance equal to one-tenth the diameter of a hydrogen molecule for sound to be heard.

The average young, healthy ear can detect sound vibrations with frequencies between approximately 16 and 16,000 Hz, although sensitivity varies greatly through this range. Maximum sensitivity is in the region of 1000 to 2000 Hz. Below 1000 Hz, sensitivity falls off dramatically. For example, to be audible, a tone with a frequency of 100 Hz must have a sound pressure 100 times greater than a tone at 1000 Hz. As most normal breath sounds are below 500 Hz, the ear is relatively insensitive to them and they are not heard as well as other types of sound (Fig 2–7).

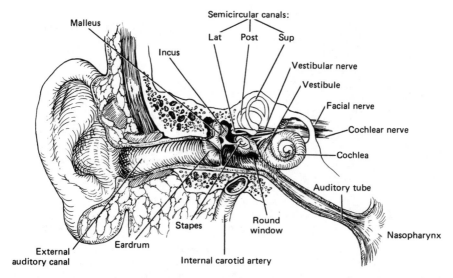

FIGURE 2-6.   The human ear. Sound waves pass through the external auditory canal inward to the tympanic membrane, or eardrum. The middle ear is an air-filled cavity in the temporal bone that opens to the outside via the auditory tube and nasopharynx, the tube usually being closed. The three ossicles—the malleus, incus, and stapes—are located in the middle ear. The manubrium, or handle, of the malleus is attached to the back of the tympanic membrane; its head is attached to the wall of the middle ear, and its short process is attached to the incus, which in turn is joined to the head of the stapes (named for its resemblance to a stirrup). The faceplate of the stapes lies against the oval window; sound waves are transmitted from here into the cochlea. Sup, superior; Post, posterior; Lat, lateral. To make the relationships clear, the cochlea has been turned slightly and the middle ear muscles have been omitted.   (From Ganong WF: *Review of Medical Physiology*. 11th ed. Los Altos, California, Lange Medical Publications, 1983. Modified and redrawn from Brödel M. *Three Unpublished Drawings of the Anatomy of the Human Ear*. Philadelphia, WB Saunders Company, 1946.)

An additional complexity of the frequency response characteristics of the ear is represented by the Fletcher–Munson phenomenon. At a high level of absolute intensity, sounds are more likely to be perceived by the ear as equally loud regardless of frequency composition. However, at a low level of absolute intensity, sounds seem to the ear to be higher pitched. The Fletcher–Munson phenomenon is not a factor when a stethoscope is being used. Yet it does affect the perception of recorded breath sounds played through a speaker; these sounds will

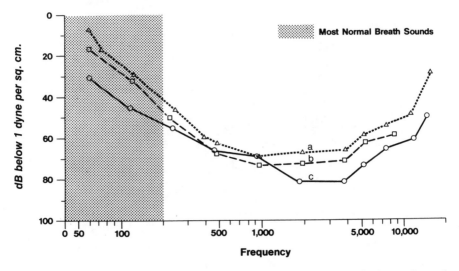

FIGURE 2-7.   *a*, Threshold sensitivity (measured in decibels or dB) of the human ear for binaural hearing in a free field. *b*, Binaural hearing in a closed system analogous to the modern stethoscope. *c*, Monaural hearing in a closed system. Note that most breath sounds fall into the range in which the ear is least sensitive.   (Modified from Wever EG, Lawrence M: *Physiological Acoustics.* Princeton, New Jersey, Princeton University Press, 1954.)

seem unnaturally low-pitched and booming to the ear when compared with breath sounds heard through a stethoscope.

Because other sensory stimuli occurring during auscultation may dull auditory perception, the examiner should see to it that interference from such stimuli is reduced to a minimum. A good clinician listening for a faint sound through the stethoscope will seek as quiet a room as possible and will also take a relaxed, comfortable position, sometimes with the eyes closed.

THE STETHOSCOPE

Since antiquity, physicians have listened to the sounds within the chest. The ancient Greeks recognized at least two characteristic sounds: (1) pleural friction rub, and (2) the splashing sound made by fluid within the chest cavity when the patient was shaken. Until the 19th century, the examiner detected these sounds by listening with the ear placed directly against the chest wall (Fig. 2-8), despite the obvious drawbacks of patients' modesty and aversion to contact.

FIGURE 2-8. Direct auscultation of the chest, portrayed in two French caricatures. (From McKusick VA: *Cardiovascular Sound in Health and Disease*. Baltimore, Williams & Wilkins, 1958.)

In 1816, a young French doctor, Rene Theophile Laennec, faced with examining the chest of a very obese woman, rolled a sheaf of paper into a cylinder; he placed one end on the patient's chest and put his ear to the other end (Fig. 2-9). Laennec named his invention the stethoscope, from the Greek *stethos*, "breast," and *skopein*, "to view." He employed subsequently a wooden cylinder, and in 1819, he published a treatise on what he had learned with his instrument. Among his metic-

FIGURE 2–9. René Théophile Laennec (1781–1826) was a French physician who invented the stethoscope and gave the first accurate descriptions of normal and abnormal breath sounds, correlating them with pathologic autopsy findings. (From Garrison FH: *An Introduction to the History of Medicine.* 4th ed. Philadelphia, WB Saunders Company, 1929, p 412.)

ulous descriptions of sounds is the following: "When the patient coughed or spoke, and still more during respiration, there was heard a tinkling like that of a small bell which has just stopped ringing or of a gnat buzzing within a porcelain vase."

The modern stethoscope is often a combination of two types of chest pieces, tubing, a binaural headset, and eartips (Fig. 2–10). These must function properly and fit well for best results. The open bell, or Ford chest piece, is similar to the old-fashioned trumpet-type hearing aid. It conducts sounds with practically no distortion. The bell is well suited for listening to low-pitched sounds. The closed diaphragm, or Bowles chest piece, has a larger diameter than the bell. The diaphragm is best suited for hearing high-pitched sounds, because it acts to attenuate low-frequency sounds and pass high-frequency sounds. But most stethoscopes tend to attenuate high frequency sounds to some degree (Charbonneau & Sudraud, 1985).

Although not outwardly apparent, the bell chest piece is converted to a diaphragm chest piece when applied too tightly to the skin. The skin acts as the diaphragm.

The binaurals should be light and comfortable. The eartubes must be inclined anteriorly in order to conform to the direction of the normal ear canals. It is impossible to overemphasize the importance of a snug yet gentle fit at the ears; the best chest piece is completely unsat-

FIGURE 2–10. Two stethoscopes in common use today. (Courtesy of Hewlett-Packard and 3M Company.)

isfactory when joined to an uncomfortable headset and poorly fitting eartips.

Broken diaphragms should not be replaced by or improvised from any odd sheet material, such as x-ray film, which is not a good diaphragm substitute. A Bowles chest piece with either a makeshift or an absent diaphragm is a very poor instrument.

The examiner should periodically inspect the tubing for deterioration and holes by flexing it (Fig. 2–11). Any damage to the tubing can render the stethoscope useless. But it is not good practice to replace the original flexible tubing with hospital tubing intended for other purposes. The manufacturer should be contacted for replacement tubing or other parts.

In 1982, Dr. John Kindig and his associates published their acoustic tests of six popular, commercially available stethoscopes. They found that, despite individual differences, there was no obviously superior model; in addition, a double-tube stethoscope held no advantage over a single-tube stethoscope. The listening ability of the examiner was far more important than the particular stethoscope being used.

(A)   (B)

FIGURE 2–11. Detecting stethoscope damage. (A) Stethoscope in unflexed position. (B) Stethoscope in flexed position. Note holes in tubing. (from Orton D, Stryker R. Sick stethoscope syndrome. *JAMA* 256:2817, 1986. Copyright 1986, American Medical Association.)

STUDY HELPS

1. What are the principal characteristics of sound? What is the significance of each characteristic?

2. What determines the quality of a sound?

3. Which breath sound is analogous to a musical note?

4. Why are breath sounds more difficult to perceive than other types of sound?

5. To what type of sound is the bell chest piece on the stethoscope well suited? To what type of sound is the diaphragm chest piece best suited?

BIBLIOGRAPHY

CHARBONNEAU G, SUDRAUD M: Mesure de la réponse en fréquence de quelques stéthoscopes usuels. Conséquences pour l'auscultation cardiaque et pulmonaire. [*Bull Eur Physiopathol Respir*] 21:49–54, 1985.

DeWEESE D, SAUNDERS WH: *Textbook of Otolaryngology.* 5th ed. St Louis, CV Mosby Company, 1977.

KINDIG JR, BEESON TP, CAMPBELL RW, et al: Acoustical performance of the stethoscope, A comparative analysis. *Am Heart J* 104:269–275, 1982.

Littmann D: Stethoscopes and auscultation. *Am J Nurs* 72:1238–1241, 1972.

McKUSICK VA: *Cardiovascular Sound in Health and Disease.* Baltimore, Williams & Wilkins, 1958.

ORTON D, STRYKER R: Sick stethoscope syndrome. *JAMA* 256:2817, 1986.

RAPPAPORT MB, SPRAGUE B: The effects of tubing bore on stethoscope efficiency. *Am Heart J* 42:605, 1951.

REISER SJ: The medical influence of the stethoscope. *Sci Am* 240(2):148–156, 1979.

3

HISTORY AND PHYSICAL EXAMINATION OF THE PATIENT WITH CHEST DISEASE

A careful history and physical examination form the basis for all diagnosis of chest disease by medical and nursing personnel. Indeed, information so obtained may be the only readily available data, particularly on a new patient or a patient seen in the home. The results will often suggest further tests that should be performed.

HISTORY

Because most patients seek medical help when they exhibit symptoms, the clinical history is likely to furnish important clues to the presence of disease. Sometimes the history alone will facilitate a prompt diagnosis; more often, it will indicate an appropriate line of investigation. A careful history must be taken, because events that seem of no significance to the patient may, in fact, be of crucial importance.

CHIEF COMPLAINT

Why is the patient seeking medical attention? What seems to be the problem (e.g., cough, shortness of breath, abnormal chest x-ray on routine physical examination)? How long has the problem existed?

FAMILY AND SOCIAL HISTORY

The family and social history of patients with pulmonary disease is important for three reasons. (1) Some infections, notably tuberculosis, are transferred from person to person; therefore, history of contact with an infected person, often an infected family member, may be elicited. (2) Allergic disorders, such as bronchial asthma, show an inherited predisposition; in addition, asthmatic attacks may be provoked by family and domestic conflict. (3) Chronic bronchitis patients may reside in a district with a high level of atmospheric pollution. However, air pollution worsens chronic bronchitis—it does not cause it.

Cigarette smoking is the most important cause of lung cancer, emphysema, and chronic bronchitis. All these conditions are quite rare in nonsmokers. The smoking history should contain the following details: (1) age at which regular smoking started, (2) average number of cigarettes or cigars smoked per day or amount of pipe tobacco consumed per week, (3) age at which smoking was terminated (if applicable). Smoking history is often recorded in terms of pack-years. For example, a man who smoked two packs of cigarettes per day for 40 years would have an 80 pack-year smoking history.

OCCUPATIONAL HISTORY

Because both acute and chronic respiratory disease may result from certain types of dust inhaled at work, a complete occupational history must cover both present and previous employment. Industrial dusts may cause respiratory disease in coal miners, stone masons, arc welders, cotton handlers, potters, steel foundry workers, and farm workers. Silica-bearing rock dust and asbestos, when inhaled, may not cause disease symptoms until years later. Thus, occupational history must contain the degree and duration of exposure to dust as well as the time relationship of such exposure to the onset of symptoms. Equally important, although not invariably occupational, are elements in the patient's environment. For example, individuals in close contact with pigeons, parrots, parakeets, or canaries may develop allergic alveolitis or psittacosis. People with a family history of allergies may develop allergic rhinitis or bronchial asthma when exposed to such allergens as pollen, house dust, feathers, animal dander, or certain fungal spores. People who live and work in a particular part of the country may be exposed to certain pulmonary disease-causing agents. An example of such an illness is coccidioidomycosis, a systemic fungal disease, respiratory in origin, that spreads via the blood to subcutaneous tissues, bone, central nervous system, and skin and other organs. Exposure to histoplasmosis, another systemic fungal disease, is common in some parts of the eastern and midwestern United States.

HISTORY OF PREVIOUS ILLNESS

In a patient with respiratory illness, valuable information may lie in the medical history, especially with regard to the following points.

TUBERCULOSIS.   Pulmonary tuberculosis in childhood may cause bronchiectasis in later life; if inadequately treated, tuberculosis may later relapse. Advanced tuberculosis of both lungs can produce severe fibrosis, leading to respiratory failure and heart failure. Bronchiectasis at the site of an inactive tuberculous lesion may be associated with the coughing up of blood. Patients should be asked about prior vaccination with bacille Calmette Guerin (BCG); when successful, this vaccination gives considerable protection against tuberculosis.

PNEUMONIA.   A few chronic pulmonary disorders, such as bronchiectasis, may begin after an episode of pneumonia, described by some patients as "pleurisy." Recurrent pneumonia, occurring in the same side of the chest, suggests bronchiectasis or lung cancer. Pneumonia is also a common problem of children with cystic fibrosis.

CHEST INJURIES AND OPERATIONS.   The circumstances of some chest injuries and operations may suggest that they are related to the present illness. For example, accidental or surgical trauma may produce a chest wall deformity. A metal foreign body, such as a bullet or shrapnel fragment, lodged in the lung may cause recurrent coughing up of blood or development of a pulmonary abscess. A traumatic hemothorax, particularly if complicated by infection, may cause gross thickening of the pleura.

PAIN

A history of chest pain frequently causes a patient to seek medical advice. The various forms of thoracic pain may be classified as follows.

PULMONARY PAIN—PRIMARY AND REFERRED.   The lung tissue and the visceral pleura covering it are insensitive to pain. Even large tumors involving these regions may cause little or no discomfort. However, pain will occur when the parietal pleura (covering the interior of the chest wall), the major airways, the chest wall, the diaphragm, or the mediastinal structures are affected by a pathologic process.

Like other forms of pain, thoracic pain may be referred to an area of skin supplied by similar nerve roots arising from the spinal cord. Thus, pain originating within the chest may cause anterior upper abdominal pain where the intercostal nerves innervate the abdominal wall. Another example is the referral of pain arising in the diaphragmatic pleura to the base of the neck and shoulder; these regions are supplied by the third, fourth, and fifth cervical nerve roots, which also make up the phrenic nerve.

Esophageal disease can cause referred thoracic pain. Esophageal spasm, achalasia, hiatus hernia, esophagitis, or carcinoma of the esophagus may be confused with cardiac and lung pathology; they all produce a similar type of pain.

PLEURAL PAIN. Acute inflammation of the parietal pleura and viral pleuritis may cause intense pain (pleurodynia). Pneumonia, pulmonary embolism, tuberculosis, and malignant disease all can cause pleuritic pain, which is localized rather than diffuse. The relationship of such pain to motions of the thorax prompts patients to describe it as a severe "catch" in the side of the chest, preventing them from breathing freely; they quickly learn that when they limit chest expansion, the pain is reduced. Motion of the trunk—bending, stooping, turning in bed—aggravates the pain; coughing and sneezing can provoke exquisite distress. Diagnostic possibilities are suggested by details of the pain history. Severe pleural pain several days after major surgery may signal a pulmonary embolus. However, the same pain associated with acute respiratory infection, fever, cough, and expectoration can indicate acute pneumonia. In a prolonged illness that is characterized by weight loss, depletion of energy, and persistent cough, pleural pain may indicate tuberculosis or chest malignancy. Pleural pain may not be distinguishable from pulmonary pain.

PAIN OF INTERCOSTAL NEURITIS. Intercostal neuritis, especially when caused by herpes zoster (shingles), may cause pain that is similar to that of pleuritis. However, neuritic pain is more likely to be superficial in character and related to coughing, sneezing, or straining but not to other movements; these characteristics are especially prominent when the neural pain is caused by a tumor of the spinal cord. The pain of intercostal neuritis is often described as an electric shock sensation, unrelated to the movements of respiration, and is sometimes associated with hypersensitive or anesthetic areas of skin on the chest wall.

MUSCULAR PAIN. Sometimes even a skilled examiner can temporarily mistake the symptoms of acute inflammation of the muscles of the chest wall, accepting them as evidence of disease within the chest. Local tenderness frequently provides a clue to the correct diagnosis.

COSTOCHONDRAL PAIN. In the condition that produces this pain, called *Tietze's syndrome*, there is tenderness on pressure and palpable enlargement of the cartilages that lie between the ribs and the sternum. Afflicted patients may fear that they have serious cardiac or pulmonary disease. The second, third, and fourth cartilages are most often affected, but any part of the large cartilaginous shield along the lower border of the thoracic cage may be involved. The pain is dull, frequently described as gnawing or aching; it bears little relationship to movement and is most noticeable when the patient is lying in bed at night. Although mild, the pain may persist for many months or years.

CARDIAC, PERICARDIAL, AND AORTIC PAIN; PAIN OF PULMONARY EMBOLUS.   Cardiac pain is in many cases so characteristic that it can be diagnosed on the basis of history alone. The patient feels it as a "crushing pain," lying beneath the sternum and to the left, radiating into the shoulders, arms, or neck. Cardiac pain caused by exertion or anxiety, relieved by rest or nitroglycerin, is typical of angina pectoris. The pain of an acutely occluded coronary artery may be confused with conditions affecting the abdomen as well as the thorax; it is retrosternal and is associated with shock, enzyme elevations, and electrocardiographic changes.

Pericardial pain, like cardiac pain, is retrosternal, extending to the left side, and, like angina, may be related to exertion. However, it is also affected by respiration and, therefore, is similar to pleural pain. Typically, the patient is relieved by sitting up and leaning forward.

Aortic pain caused by an aneurysm, especially a dissecting one, is described by the patient as a deep, boring, agonizing, tearing pain; it may be compared to the pain of a severe toothache. The location is retrosternal or, sometimes, interscapular.

Pulmonary embolus may sometimes produce pain along with shortness of breath, hemoptysis (rarely), and cough.

COUGH

Cough is a cardinal sign of pulmonary disease. Secretions of the bronchial mucosa are constantly produced and flow in an orderly manner from smaller to larger airways; they are propelled by tiny, finger-like structures called cilia. Finally, they ascend the trachea, mix with saliva, and are swallowed. In normal people, all this is accomplished without cough. Therefore, any cough suggests an abnormality—possibly trivial, perhaps critical.

There are basically two types of cough: productive and nonproductive. A productive cough clears the airways of the viscous secretions that accumulate in many pulmonary disorders. Nonproductive cough is an irritative phenomenon and serves no useful purpose; the stimulus for it may be mechanical or chemical, including inflammatory reactions.

A loose cough, accompanied by a low-pitched, rattling sound, is often associated with heavy smoking habits, history of bronchitis, copious daily sputum volume, and relatively poor performance in forced expiratory tests. The source of the rattling sound is presumably the passage of gas through airways that are lightly occluded.

The type of sputum produced is suggestive of the pathologic process. Foul-smelling sputum is often found in anaerobic bacterial infection—lung abscess, for example. Abundant, frothy, saliva-like sputum is a rare but characteristic symptom of bronchioloalveolar carcinoma. Voluminous, pink, frothy sputum is seen in patients with pulmonary edema. Pneumococcal pneumonia is often associated with rust-colored sputum. Copious purulent sputum, brought up on change of posture, may indicate bronchiectasis.

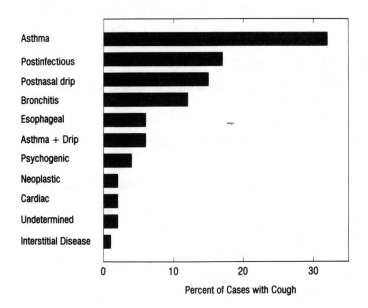

FIGURE 3–1. Causes of chronic cough in two series of patients (158 patients total). Percentage does not equal one hundred because of rounding of numbers. (From Irwin RS, Corrao WM, Pratter, MR: Chronic persistent cough in the adult: The spectrum and frequency of causes and successful outcome of specific therapy. *Am Rev Resp Dis* 123:413–417, 1981; and from Poe RH, Israel RH, Utell MJ, Hall WJ: Chronic cough: Bronchoscopy or pulmonary function testing? *Am Rev Resp Dis* 126:160–162, 1982. Data tabulated in Murray JF: Diagnostic evaluation. History and physical examination. In *Textbook of Respiratory Medicine*. Murray JF, Nadel, JA (eds). Philadelphia, WB Saunders Company, 1988, Table 25–1, p 434.)

At times, severe episodes of coughing can progress to muscular exhaustion and unconsciousness, called cough syncope. This condition is usually found in strong, middle-aged men who smoke excessively. Chronic bronchitis and asthma are frequently also present. Although the cause is unknown, hyperventilation with excessive loss of carbon dioxide from the blood is suspected.

Figure 3–1 shows causes of cough in two series of patients.

HEMOPTYSIS

Hemoptysis, the coughing up of blood, is a frightening experience that usually causes a patient to seek medical advice without delay. Small streaks of blood may appear in the sputum of patients with acute respiratory tract infections; grossly bloody sputum may be coughed up by

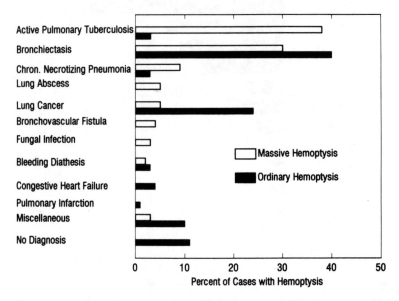

FIGURE 3–2. Comparison of causes of "ordinary" and "massive" hemoptysis from two recent series of 129 and 123 patients, respectively. (From Gong H, Salvatierra C: Clinical efficacy of early and delayed fiberoptic bronchoscopy in patients with hemoptysis. *Am Rev Resp Dis* 124:221–225, 1981; and from Conlan AA, Hurwitz SS, Kriege L, Nicolaou N, Pool R. Massive hemoptysis. Review of 123 cases. *J Thorac Cardiovasc Surg* 85:120–124, 1983. Data tabulated in Murray JF: Diagnostic evaluation. History and physical examination. In *Textbook of Respiratory Medicine.* Murray JF, Nadel JA, (eds). Philadelphia, WB Saunders Company, 1988, Table 25–2, p 435.)

TABLE 3–1. Differential Diagnosis of Hemoptysis and Hematemesis.*

Feature	Hemoptysis	Hematemesis
Prodrome	Tingling in throat, desire to cough	Nausea, stomach distress
Onset	Blood is coughed up; retching may accompany	Blood is vomited; coughing may accompany
Appearance	Some portions frothy	Never frothy
Color	Portions may be bright red	Uniformly dark red
pH reaction	Alkaline	Acid
Content	Leukocytes, microorganisms, hemosiderin-laden macrophages	Food particles
Past history	Lung disease	Alcoholism, peptic ulcer, liver disease
Anemia	Occasionally present	Common
Stools (at onset)	Guaiac negative	Guaiac positive

*From Hinshaw HC, Murray JF: *Diseases of the Chest*, 4th ed. Philadelphia, WB Saunders Company, 1980, p. 11. Used by permission.

patients with pneumonia. Some patients who expectorate bloody sputum are seriously ill; they may have bronchiectasis, tuberculosis, mitral stenosis, or bronchogenic carcinoma. Most commonly, they have bronchitis.

In many cases, the patient is not aware of the origin of the blood. He will commonly state that it just "welled up" in his throat. Although the blood may occasionally come from a source in the nasopharynx, most commonly it originates either from the gastrointestinal tract (hematemesis) or from the lung.

Bleeding from esophageal varices may be confused with hemoptysis. Usually, however, blood is vomited during variceal bleeding, and the patient subsequently notes black stools. Other features distinguishing hemoptysis from hematemesis are noted in Table 3–1. Figure 3–2 shows a comparison of "ordinary" and massive hemoptysis from two recent series.

DYSPNEA

Dyspnea, or difficult breathing, is most often described by patients as shortness of breath. Because breathing is such a primitive, urgent human need, dyspnea is more profoundly disturbing to the patient than almost any other symptom.

Circumstances associated with the dyspnea should be carefully noted by the examiner. Is the dyspnea associated with exertion? Does it occur after the patient walks half a block or climbs one flight of stairs? Dyspnea accompanied by wheezing may result from exercise-induced asthma. Although paroxysmal nocturnal dyspnea is a sign of left ventricular failure, it may sometimes be confused with bronchial asthma. Sudden, unprovoked dyspnea may result from spontaneous pneumothorax, pulmonary embolism, or myocardial infarction. Many patients with advanced lung disease also complain of paroxysmal nocturnal dyspnea and orthopnea.

In addition, the emotional state of the patient must be taken into account; shortness of breath, not related to exertion and not caused by organic disease but associated with anxiety states, is a common complaint. The patient will say that the air "doesn't go deep enough," that he can't get enough air, and that the sense of air hunger is difficult to relieve, even with deep, sighing breaths. During the interview, the irregular breathing habits and occasional deep sighs will be apparent to the examiner. Although the diagnosis is usually obvious, a thorough examination, including pulmonary function tests, should be performed.

Some very emotional patients with psychogenic air hunger will hyperventilate, reducing dissolved arterial carbon dioxide below normal. This condition is encountered frequently. The increasingly forceful, rapid breathing is followed by numbness of the extremities, tingling sensations around the mouth, and mild clouding of consciousness, but rarely complete syncope. The diagnosis is made by asking the patient to breathe deeply and rapidly for 1 to 2 minutes and then to compare the symptoms produced with those that occur during spontaneous attacks.

HOARSENESS AND WHEEZE

Hoarseness is usually due to an abnormality of the larynx and vocal cords. Occasionally, however, hoarseness may be the result of a lung tumor or aortic aneurysm that damages the recurrent laryngeal nerve, resulting in left vocal cord paralysis.

When a patient complains of wheeze, he may have various conditions in mind. Some people use wheeze to describe noisy and labored breathing; others apply it to rattling secretions in the upper airways. However, wheeze usually denotes the musical sounds that are described more fully in Chapter 5. Many patients become so accustomed to wheezing that they cease to be aware of it unless it is called to their attention. The patient should be asked when the wheeze is present and whether it is made worse by exertion, inhalation of dust, or a respiratory infection.

Some patients with stridor, which is discussed fully in Chapter 5, may describe it as a wheeze. Care must be taken to differentiate between these two sounds. Stridor, a high-pitched musical or "crowing" sound, usually results from obstruction of a major airway; it demands urgent investigation and treatment.

PHYSICAL EXAMINATION

Every examiner should develop a routine, a specific sequence in which the procedures of physical examination—inspection, palpation, percussion, and auscultation—are performed. The learning of a routine will assure that no aspect of the examination is forgotten. Usually, the blood pressure is measured first, after which the heart rate is determined while a thermometer is in the patient's mouth to register body temperature. The remainder of the examination may then proceed.

INSPECTION

To begin, the patient should be unclothed to the waist. The room should be well lighted. Above all, both the patient and the examiner should be in a comfortable position; if either is uncomfortable, the examination will be hurried and, as a consequence, less thorough.

The examiner should first note whether the patient is breathless when talking or whether he or she is able to articulate long sentences without stopping to breathe. Hoarseness and stridor should be obvious at this time. Normal breathing is quiet except for occasional sighs; audible wheezing indicates severe bronchospasm. The gurgling of secretions suggests mucus retention; endotracheal suction may be necessary.

Observation of the sputum is mandatory. It should be inspected for color, odor, and the presence of mucous plugs. If a cup is present at the bedside, the amount produced over 24 hours should be noted; any increase may suggest a worsening of the patient's condition.

If the patient is coughing, the nature of the cough should be noted. A weak cough may be due to weakness or paralysis of respiratory muscles, anesthesia, or use of sedatives or narcotics. Patients with a weak cough are prone to mucus retention, atelectasis, and abnormal blood gas levels because of their inability to cough up secretions. A dry, hacking cough suggests airway irritation.

SKIN COLOR. The skin, mucous membranes, conjunctiva, soft palate, lips, and tongue should be observed to detect cyanosis and pallor. Cyanosis is a bluish or grayish tinge to the skin that is caused by diminished oxygen content of the blood; when especially marked, cyanosis may indicate impending cardiorespiratory collapse. Pallor, a paleness of the skin, may indicate anemia or chronic illness; however, some healthy people are normally quite pale. In advanced pulmonary disease, patients may develop a reddish-blue tint to the skin, the result of increased total hemoglobin and increased unoxygenated hemoglobin.

NECK VEIN DISTENTION.   In chronic obstructive pulmonary disease, the neck veins distend on expiration and collapse on inspiration, especially in a very breathless patient. Expiratory distention is the result of positive pressure in the chest from increased work of breathing; inspiratory collapse occurs as negative pressure within the thorax facilitates the return of venous blood to the heart. If the patient has right ventricular heart failure as well as pulmonary disease, the inspiratory collapse may not occur.

EXTREMITIES.   The fingers and fingernails should be examined for evidence of clubbing and tobacco stains. Clubbing, an abnormality of the nails and distal phalanges, causes bulbous changes of the fingertips (Fig. 3–3) and toes. Although clubbing may be a normal familial trait, it is often seen in patients with congenital heart disease,

FIGURE 3–3.   Top view of the right hand and side view of the index finger of a patient with advanced clubbing resulting from interstitial lung disease.   (From Hinshaw HC, Murray JF: *Diseases of the Chest.* 4th ed. Philadelphia, WB Saunders Company, 1980, p 21.)

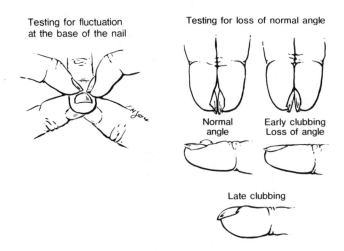

Testing for fluctuation at the base of the nail

Testing for loss of normal angle

Normal angle

Early clubbing Loss of angle

Late clubbing

FIGURE 3–4.   Signs of and tests for clubbing.

subacute bacterial endocarditis, bronchiectasis, cystic fibrosis, lung abscess, pulmonary fibrosis, lung cancer, liver cirrhosis, chronic ulcerative colitis, and regional enteritis.

Early clubbing can be detected by noting whether or not the normal slight angle is present between the nail and the finger (Fig. 3–4). In early clubbing, this angle is lost, and the base of the nail bed will feel soft and spongy. As the condition progresses, the nail feels as though it is floating in a bed of soft vascular tissue. In advanced clubbing, the nail takes on a so-called watch glass deformity, and the fingertips become wider and rounder; the overlying skin stretches, loses normal wrinkles, and has a polished, glistening appearance.

Hypertrophic pulmonary osteoarthropathy is characterized pathologically by bilateral subperiosteal bone formation along long and tubular bones. Deformity of the digits will be associated with enlarged ankles, wrists, interphalangeal joints of the fingers and toes, and distal ends of the long bones in the arms and legs. This condition is most common in lung cancer.

EXAMINATION OF THE CHEST WALL

In order to describe abnormalities of the chest, the examiner should be aware of certain anatomic reference points (Fig. 3–5). The suprasternal notch marks the top point of the manubrium. The sternal angle is the point at which the manubrium and body of the sternum join; the anterior portion of the second rib also attaches here. Figure 3–6 shows the following additional anatomic reference points.

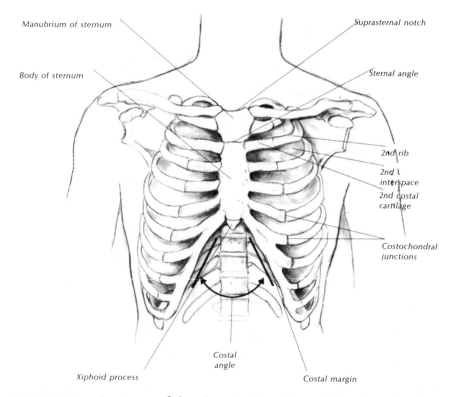

FIGURE 3–5.   Anatomy of the chest wall.   (From Bates B: *A Guide to Physical Examination*. Philadelphia, JB Lippincott Company, 1974, p 173.)

Midsternal line: a line extending downward from the sternal notch.

Midclavicular line: a vertical line parallel to the midsternal line and extending downward from the midpoint of each clavicle.

Anterior axillary line: a line extending downward from the anterior axillary fold.

Posterior axillary line: a line parallel to the anterior axillary line beginning at the posterior axillary fold.

Midaxillary line: a vertical line starting at a point midway between the anterior and posterior axillary lines.

Midspinal line: a vertical line in the center of the back running along the spinal processes.

Midscapular lines: vertical lines on the back, parallel to the midspinal line, extending through the apices of the scapulae.

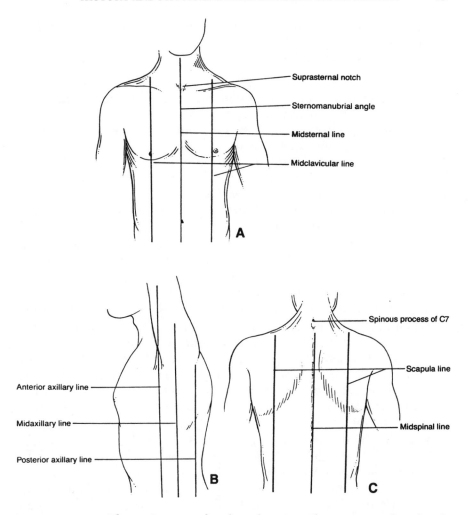

FIGURE 3-6. Thoracic cage landmarks. (*A*) The topographic landmarks of the anterior thorax. (*B*) The landmarks on the lateral view. (*C*) The landmarks of the posterior thorax. (From Swartz MH: *Textbook of Physical Diagnosis*. Philadelphia, WB Saunders Company, 1989, pp 210–211.)

Infrascapular area: area of the posterior thorax lying below the scapulae.

Interscapular area: area of the posterior thorax lying between the scapulae.

Using these landmarks, the examiner should record the site of an identifying mark, percussion abnormality, auscultatory sound, or other change as, for example, "5 cm to the right of the midsternal line at the level of the fourth rib."

Certain abnormalities in the shape of the chest should be noted (Fig. 3–7).

1. Increase in anteroposterior diameter relative to lateral diameter. This ratio varies in normal people from about 5:7 to 1:2. However, in patients with chronic obstructive pulmonary disease, primarily emphysema, the anteroposterior dimension of the chest may increase to such an extent that the ratio of the two dimensions approximates 1:1, a condition referred to as barrel chest. Care should be taken to distinguish barrel chest from kyphosis, an abnormally increased curvature of the spine that also increases the anteroposterior diameter.

2. Pectus carinatum, or "pigeon breast," is commonly the result of chronic respiratory disease in childhood. It is characterized by a localized prominence of the sternum and adjacent rib cartilages, often associated with indrawn ribs forming symmetric horizontal grooves (Harrison's sulci) above the usually everted rib margins.

3. Pectus excavatum, or "funnel chest," is a congenital abnormality, a localized depression of the lower end of the sternum, or, uncommonly, depression of the entire sternum and the attached rib cartilages. Pectus excavatum generally is asymptomatic; however, when severe, the ventilatory capacity of the lungs may be diminished, accompanied by heart murmurs and other disturbances in cardiac function.

4. Kyphosis, an increase in the normal curvature of the thoracic spine, causes the patient to appear hunched over or hunchbacked. Although now frequently associated with the osteoporosis of the aging process, kyphosis is also seen in spinal tuberculosis (Pott's disease); it results from the inflammation-induced vertebral deformity. Kyphosis appears in people with rheumatoid arthritis, Paget's disease, acromegaly, or many years of poor posture.

    Kyphosis, although usually an increased curvature of the spine, may also appear in the form of an *angular kyphosis*—a protruding hump in the back resulting from the collapse of one or more vertebral bodies. The hump, called a *gibbus*, may accompany tuberculosis of the spine or any other condition producing compression fractures of the vertebrae.

5. Scoliosis is a lateral curvature of the thoracic spine, accompanied by vertebral rotation. The disc spaces become narrower on the concave side of the curve and wider on the convex side. The vertebral bodies become wedged and are thicker on the convex side. In most cases of scoliosis, called idiopathic scoliosis, the cause is

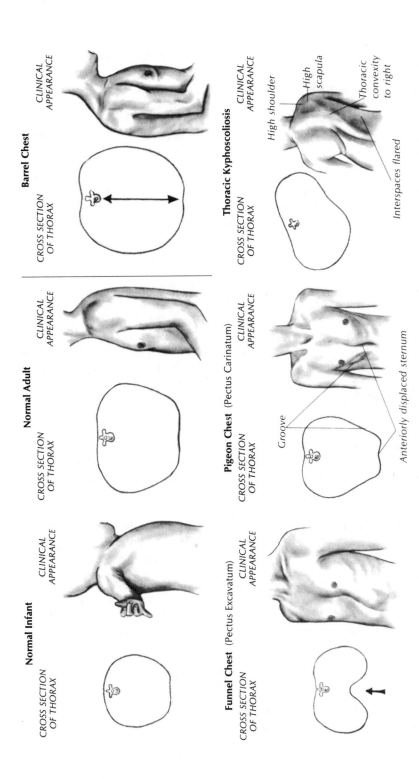

Normal Infant

CROSS SECTION OF THORAX

CLINICAL APPEARANCE

Normal Adult

CROSS SECTION OF THORAX

CLINICAL APPEARANCE

Barrel Chest

CROSS SECTION OF THORAX

CLINICAL APPEARANCE

Funnel Chest (Pectus Excavatum)

CROSS SECTION OF THORAX

CLINICAL APPEARANCE

Pigeon Chest (Pectus Carinatum)

CROSS SECTION OF THORAX

CLINICAL APPEARANCE

Groove

Anteriorly displaced sternum

Thoracic Kyphoscoliosis

CROSS SECTION OF THORAX

CLINICAL APPEARANCE

High shoulder

High scapula

Thoracic convexity to right

Interspaces flared

FIGURE 3-7. Deformities of the thorax. (From Bates: *A Guide to Physical Examination*. Philadelphia, JB Lippincott Company, 1974, p 93.)

45

unknown, although about 90 percent of these are genetic and hereditary. Some cases are caused by congenital vertebral deformity, poliomyelitis, neurofibromatosis, or juvenile rheumatoid arthritis. Idiopathic scoliosis occurs approximately seven times more often in girls than in boys. It is classified as infantile, juvenile, and adult types, according to well-defined peak periods of onset.

Infantile idiopathic scoliosis begins between birth and 3 years of age. It is more common in males, and the majority of cases resolve spontaneously, even if not treated.

Juvenile idiopathic scoliosis occurs between the ages of 4 and 10 years. It is more evenly distributed between the sexes, most cases being recognized when the patient is about 6 years old.

Adolescent idiopathic scoliosis consists of those cases diagnosed between the age of 10 years and skeletal maturity. Seventy percent of affected children are girls. In general, all cases of scoliosis tend to progress most rapidly during the years of adolescent growth.

In mild cases of scoliosis, there is a single lateral curve, usually toward the right. In more severe cases, there is a thoracic curve and a compensatory lumbar curve, causing an S- or backward S-shaped deformity of the spine. Severe scoliosis is readily apparent in the standing patient. Milder cases can be identified by the elevated shoulder and humping of ribs on one side of the back when the patient bends forward.

Scoliosis is a significant finding in the patient with chest disease because of the respiratory impairment associated with severe spinal deformity. The curvature and rotation of the spine cause advancing respiratory restriction later in life; these patients may die of severe pneumonia superimposed on the preexisting respiratory impairment.

In all advanced cases of scoliosis, breath sounds will be diminished on the side of the chest in which the ribs are crowded together, reflecting the poor alveolar ventilation and air flow.

6. Kyphoscoliosis is a combination of backward and lateral curvature of the spine. Of all spinal deformities, this one causes the most serious physical impairment of the heart and lungs. Many patients have severe cardiac and respiratory failure by middle age.

In addition to the above-noted abnormalities in the shape of the chest, certain chest wall lesions should also be mentioned.

1. Skin abnormalities—eruptions, nodules, purple spots or bruises, scars of surgery or trauma.

2. Subcutaneous changes—particularly swellings. Subcutaneous emphysema, the presence of air in the subcutaneous tissues, may

result in diffuse swelling of the chest wall, the neck, and, uncommonly, the face. The air-filled tissues have a characteristic crackling sensation when palpated. Subcutaneous emphysema of the chest usually occurs when air from a tension pneumothorax escapes along the track of a needle or catheter used to decompress the pleural space. When alveoli rupture, air can also escape into the mediastinum, causing mediastinal emphysema.

3. Other chest wall abnormalities—spider telangiectases (dilatation of small vessels) in liver disease; enlarged blood vessels (veins in superior vena cava syndrome, arteries in coarctation of the aorta); localized prominences and bone deformities.

Tracheal position should be midline; this will be discussed more fully in the section on palpation.

OBSERVATION OF RESPIRATORY MOTIONS

A normal adult takes about 14 breaths per minute. While the subject is breathing quietly, the examiner should observe the chest wall for symmetric bilateral expansion; this observation is best made with the subject lying supine and the examiner watching from the foot of the bed. If there is asymmetry, decreased size, or restricted expansion of one side of the thorax, disease may be present: for example, thickened fibrotic pleura, pleural inflammation, or trauma such as a fractured rib.

If the patient is breathing abnormally, the examiner should record the exact abnormality. *Bradypnea*, an abnormal slowing of respiration, may result from oxygen toxicity, primary hypoventilation, opiates, or brain tumor. *Apnea* is a temporary cessation of respiration. *Tachypnea*, an increased respiratory rate, may be seen in fever, pneumonia, or metabolic alkalosis; it is also seen in anxiety states and after exercise. *Hyperpnea*, an increase in the depth of respiration, is sometimes called air hunger and is frequently associated with metabolic acidosis. *Periodic respiration*, which is alternating hyperpnea and apnea, may be present in relatively serious disease states, although it is occasionally observed as a non-pathologic occurrence in the child and in the normal sleeping adult.

One variant of periodic respiration, Cheyne–Stokes breathing, was originally described in a case report by John Cheyne himself as follows: "His breathing was irregular; it would entirely cease for a quarter of a minute, then it would become perceptible, though very low, then by degrees it became heaving and quick, and then it would gradually cease again. This revolution in the state of his breathing occupied about a minute, during which there were about 30 acts of respiration." This form of breathing takes place when the brain's respiratory center in the medulla and the regulating corticobulbar tracts lose their usual fine sensitivity to fluctuations in carbon dioxide tension or nervous stimuli; it is most common in cerebral disorders such as cerebrovascular accidents; it is also seen in brain tumor, heart disease, chronic kidney disease, meningitis, and pneumonia.

A striking form of abnormal breathing, Biot's respiration, may be seen in meningitis and medullary lesions. Camille Biot first described it as follows: "This irregularity of the respiratory movements is not periodic, sometimes slow, sometimes rapid, sometimes superficial, sometimes deep, but without any constant relation of succession between the two types, with pauses following irregular intervals, preceded and often followed by a sigh more or less prolonged."

Another abnormal breathing pattern is *sighing respiration*. Sighing respiration is characterized by deep inspiration interrupting the normal respiratory rhythm, often accompanied by an audible sigh. This form of breathing is almost always a sign of emotional tension and is rarely associated with organic disease. Spirograms of some of the breathing patterns described here are presented in Figure 3–8.

Besides respiratory rhythm, pulmonary disease may affect the mode of breathing. In normal people, as was mentioned in Chapter 1, inspiration is mediated by contraction of the external intercostal muscles and the diaphragm, whereas expiration is passive, dependent on the elastic recoil of the lungs. Women tend to use the intercostal muscles, whereas men and infants of both sexes use the diaphragm. The following departures from the norm should be recorded.

1. If the mode of breathing is exclusively thoracic and confined to the intercostal muscles, the examiner should suspect that diaphragmatic movement is inhibited by the following: (a) peritoneal irritation; (b) severe abdominal distention from ascites, gaseous distention of the bowel, a large ovarian cyst, or pregnancy; or (c) diaphragmatic paralysis.

2. If the mode of breathing is exclusively abdominal, lack of chest expansion may be due to ankylosing spondylitis, intercostal paralysis, or pleural pain.

As was mentioned in Chapter 1, patients use the accessory muscles of respiration—sternocleidomastoids, scaleni, and trapezii—when pulmonary function is compromised and adequate ventilation is not possible. These muscles lift the ribs out and up with every breath and are utilized in such conditions as advanced emphysema, severe bronchial asthma, and obstruction of the larynx and trachea. Moreover, such breathing is often accompanied by retraction of the suprasternal and supraclavicular fossae, the intercostal spaces, and the epigastrium with each inspiration.

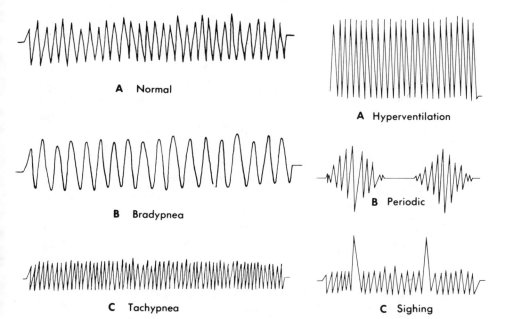

FIGURE 3-8.   Spirograms of normal, slow, and rapid respiration (left), and altered respiration (right).   (From Prior JA: Thorax and Lungs. In Prior JA, Silberstein JS, Stang JM: *Physical Diagnosis*. 6th ed. St. Louis, CV Mosby Company, 1981.)

Even more retraction of the chest wall is present in patients who have sustained a series of double fractures of the ribs or sternum (flail chest). The region of chest wall between the fractures becomes mobile and is sucked in with each inspiration. This *paradoxical movement* gravely hampers pulmonary ventilation and thus may be accompanied by severe respiratory distress and hypoxia.

In addition to the abnormal inspiratory movements already described, abnormal expiratory movements may result from strong contractions of the abdominal muscles and latissimus dorsi, particularly if elastic recoil of the lungs is not sufficient to fully expel air from the alveoli. These abnormal expiratory movements are seen in some types of emphysema or in cases in which expiratory airway obstruction is present—bronchial asthma and some forms of chronic bronchitis, for example. Patients so afflicted sit upright, holding the bed table or back of chair, fixing the shoulder girdle so that the latissimus dorsi can be used to approximate the ribs and augment the respiratory effort. These patients purse their lips during expiration to keep the intrabronchial pressure above that in the adjacent alveoli, preventing collapse of the bronchial walls.

FIGURE 3–9.   Lymph node regions of the neck. (*1*) Preauricular—in front of the ear; (*2*) posterior auricular—superficial to the mastoid process; (*3*) occipital—at the base of the skull posteriorly; (*4*) tonsillar—at the angle of the mandible; (*5*) submaxillary—halfway between the angle and the tip of the mandible; (*6*) submental—in the midline behind the tip of the mandible; (*7*) superficial cervical—superficial to the sternomastoid; (*8*) posterior cervical chain—along the anterior edge of the trapezius; (*9*) deep cervical chain—deeper than the sternomastoid and often inaccessible to examination. To find these lymph nodes, the examiner hooks the thumb and fingers around either side of the sternomastoid muscle; (*10*) supraclavicular—deep in the angle formed by the clavicle and sternomastoid. (From Bates B: *A Guide to Physical Examination*. Philadelphia, JB Lippincott Company, 1974, p 45.)

PALPATION

A considerable amount of information pertinent to the thorax and lungs can be gathered by palpation; the knowledge gained by history and inspection may be supplemented.

One of the most important functions of palpation is the careful search for lymph nodes. The examiner should palpate the cervical nodal chains and the supraclavicular regions on both sides, rolling the skin over underlying structures, first lightly, then more heavily, to locate any nodes, superficial or deep. Even the smallest node may prove to be of paramount significance; biopsy of such a node may be the only practical means of making a diagnosis of lung cancer (Fig. 3–9).

The axillary nodes should be examined with great care. The examiner should bear the weight of the patient's relaxed arm; one hand is then placed at the elbow, the other reaches high into the axillary space. The group of nodes usually found in this region should be rolled under the fingers.

The trachea is palpated to detect any deviation from its normal position in the middle of the neck. If one lung is atelectatic, the trachea will be displaced to the side of the abnormality, particularly on inspi-

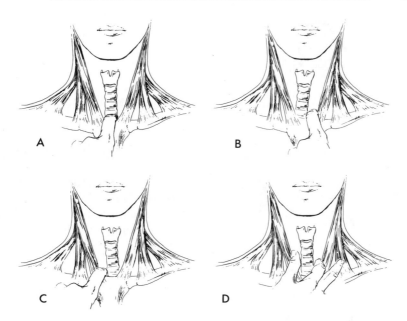

FIGURE 3–10.   Determining the position of the trachea. (*A*) With the patient's neck flexed and chin in the midline position, check for anterior displacement of the trachea (shallow suprasternal notch) by inserting fingertip directly in the middle of the suprasternal notch. Inability to place a fingertip into this notch indicates anterior displacement. (*B*) and (*C*) Check for lateral displacement of the trachea by firmly inserting the index finger in the suprasternal notch, first on the left side and then on the right. The spaces should feel symmetrical. (*D*) Some clinicians prefer to check for tracheal deviation by palpating with the thumb and forefinger.

ration (Fig. 3–10). Fixed lateral displacement of the trachea may be the result of aortic aneurysm, mediastinal tumor, neck tumor, unilaterally enlarged paratracheal lymph nodes, or unilateral thyroid enlargement. The trachea will deviate on expiration from the affected hemithorax in tension pneumothorax, large hemothorax, or pleural effusion. Anterior displacement of the trachea, indicated by a suprasternal notch into which a fingertip cannot be inserted, is seen in tumor behind the trachea, some cases of goiter, and dilated esophagus in achalasia. Palpable voice-generated vibrations transmitted to the chest wall are called *tactile fremitus* or *vocal fremitus*. To elicit this sign, the examiner asks the patient to count "one, two, three" or say "ninety-nine." The palpating hand is placed, palm against the chest, on equivalent areas of the chest wall, that is, over equivalent bronchopulmonary segments, on either side of the chest. Vocal fremitus is most intense in the slender adult

FIGURE 3–11. Respiratory motion of the rib margins. The examiner should watch for the excursion of his thumbs and feel for the range and symmetry of respiratory movement. (From Bates B: *A Guide to Physical Examination*. Philadelphia, JB Lippincott Company, 1974, p 82.)

male, less intense in women. Increased fremitus on one side indicates that sound is being transmitted better through a more solid, less aerated lung and suggests tissue consolidation, often a result of lobar pneumonia. Decreased or absent fremitus, the result of conditions that favor less sound transmission, may occur when there is fibrous thickening of the pleura, when fluid is present in the pleural space, or when there is air in the pleural space (pneumothorax).

Respiratory motion of the rib margins can be gauged by palpation. The sides of the chest are grasped firmly, as in Figure 3–11. The hands should be placed so that there is a loose fold of skin between the two thumbs, which can then move apart as the chest expands. The movement of the thumbs serves as an accurate gauge of the relative movement of the two sides of the chest.

PERCUSSION

Percussion is the tapping of body structures to produce a sound. Two methods of percussion are employed over the chest: (1) *immediate percussion*, during which the examiner strikes the chest with either the palmar aspect of the middle finger or the tips of four fingers held tightly together; and (2) *mediate percussion*, during which the examiner holds a solid object, called the pleximeter (commonly the middle finger),

A   **B**

FIGURE 3-12. Immediate percussion with the middle finger. (*A*) The finger poised to strike the chest wall. (*B*) The palmar aspect of the finger striking the chest wall. (From Prior JA: Thorax and lungs. In Prior JA, Silberstein JS, Stang JM: *Physical Diagnosis*. 6th ed. St. Louis, CV Mosby Company, 1981.)

against the chest; a second object, the plexor (usually the middle finger of the other hand), strikes the pleximeter, generating a sound (Figs. 3–12 and 3–13). As in the evaluation of vocal fremitus, the percussion sound from one side of the chest should be compared with the sound on the opposite side. Percussion is generally performed at the following sites: (1) the midportion of each clavicle; (2) the lung apices; (3) the posterior thorax at several points from the apices to the bases of the lungs; (4) the axillary and midaxillary regions; and (5) the anterior portion of the chest (see Fig. 4–1).

The percussion sounds vary considerably in quality in different subjects and over different parts of the chest. The sounds generated over a normal lung are often described as *resonant*. Notes of short duration and low intensity, normally found over the liver and the heart, are called *dull*. High-pitched sounds, such as those over the air-containing stomach, are called *tympanitic* (Fig. 3–14).

Pathologic changes in the chest will alter the percussion sounds. When percussion is performed over an area of pneumonic consolidation, the sound evoked will be dull rather than resonant. Percussion over an emphysematous lung or a pneumothorax will produce a deep, sustained *hyperresonant* sound.

Percussion may be used to determine whether position and motion of the diaphragms are normal. First, the patient is told to take

A   B

FIGURE 3–13.   Mediate percussion. (*A*) The wrist is cocked and ready to strike. (*B*) The plexor fingertip is striking the pleximeter finger. Only the pleximeter finger touches the patient's back.   (From Prior JA: Thorax and lungs. In Prior JA, Silberstein JS, Stang JM: *Physical Diagnosis*. 6th ed. St. Louis, CV Mosby Company, 1981.)

a deep breath and hold it. Second, the lower margin of resonance, which represents the level of the diaphragm, is determined by percussion; in doing so, the examiner moves the pleximeter finger downward until a definite change in tonal quality is heard. Third, the patient is instructed to exhale as far as possible and hold his breath; percussion is then repeated. The distance between the two levels indicates the range of motion of the diaphragm, normally about 3 to 5 cm (Fig. 3–15). The diaphragmatic excursion will be reduced in patients with severe emphysema, pleural inflammation, and splinting due to pain. In carcinoma of the lung, when the phrenic nerve has been damaged, diaphragmatic motion on one side may be absent. In addition, diaphragmatic excursion cannot be assessed in the presence of pleural effusion.

Percussion over the clavicles, a valuable technique in detecting lesions of the upper lobes, differs from that used elsewhere. The clavicles should be percussed directly with the right middle finger or with

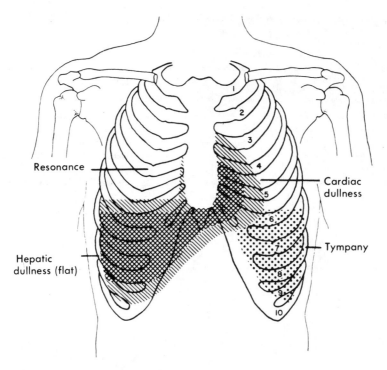

FIGURE 3–14.   Regions over the normal thorax where resonance, dull-ness, and tympany are elicited during percussion.   (From Prior JA: Thorax and lungs. In Prior JA, Silberstein JS, Stang JM: *Physical Diag-nosis.* 6th ed. St. Louis, CV Mosby Company, 1981.)

the right index, middle, and ring fingers held closely together. The medial third of the clavicle, just lateral to its enlarged medial end, will yield the best diagnostic information. Percussion more laterally will simply elicit dullness from the muscle masses of the shoulder. Auscul-tation is discussed in Chapter 4.

Auscultatory percussion. During this procedure, the examiner taps his finger gently over the manubrium of the sternum, while listen-ing over the posterior chest wall with a stethoscope. A decrease in sound amplitude is ascribed to a lung abnormality. Some clinicians believe that auscultatory percussion is capable of identifying pulmo-nary lesions deep within the chest. However, one recent study suggests that the sound of the percussion travels mainly through chest wall structures, not through lung tissue. Therefore, the usefulness of aus-cultatory percussion in detecting deep chest lesions is highly question-able (Bohadana et al., 1989).

FIGURE 3–15. Normal range of diaphragmatic motion detectable by percussion. (From Prior JA: Thorax and lungs. In Prior JA, Silberstein JS, Stang JM: *Physical Diagnosis.* 6th ed. St. Louis, CV Mosby Company, 1981, p 191.)

CLINICAL AND LABORATORY TESTS FOR PATHOLOGIC CONDITIONS

RADIOGRAPHIC EXAMINATION. *Posteroanterior* and *lateral radiographs* of the chest may reveal a lesion that was undetected by history and physical examination, may show its position, and may sometimes suggest a pathologic condition. *Chest fluoroscopy* provides information regarding mobility of the diaphragm, which is of particular importance in lung cancer. For example, if one side of the diaphragm is paralyzed, the tumor has probably damaged the phrenic nerve. *Tomography* (Fig. 3–16) is a radiographic technique capable of visualizing an opacity or abnormality lying in one particular anatomic plane; the opacity may have been obscured by overlying structures in the ordinary radiograph. Tomography is of particular value in locating lung cavities and flecks of calcium in a lung lesion and in defining irregular densities. *Pulmonary angiography* (Fig. 3–17) can be used to differentiate solid chest masses from blood vessels or to detect vascular obstruction. A pulmonary angiogram is made by taking films in quick succession after injecting contrast medium into the main pulmonary artery. *Computerized axial tomography (CT scanning)* employs x-rays and a computer to reconstruct very detailed cross-sectional images.

FIGURE 3–16.   Cavity rendered more visible by tomography. Large cavity in right upper lobe that is barely visible in the routine film (*A*). Tomogram (*B*) reveals the borders of the cavity with greater clarity. Conventional chest films are made at 2 m, whereas tomograms are made at 1 m or less; there is therefore increased magnification in the latter. (From Hinshaw HC, Murray JF: *Diseases of the Chest.* 4th ed. Philadelphia, WB Saunders Company, 1981, p 45.)

This technique provides an additional dimension to conventional radiography and helps to clarify or identify lesions not clearly visualized by other methods.

RADIOISOTOPE SCANNING.   Perfusion scans of the lung are done by injecting intravenously the radioactive compound technetium 99m (99m-Tc)-labeled microspheres (Fig. 3–18). These tiny, biodegradable particles are trapped in the lung tissue. The radiation they emit is collected by a device called a gamma camera, which creates an image of the perfused tissue. A second type of scan, a ventilation study, performed by allowing the patient to inhale radioactive xenon gas, can be compared with the perfusion study to diagnose pulmonary embolus (Fig. 3–19). For example, if a section of lung is ventilated but not perfused, an embolus is probably present. But if a section of lung is both unventilated and unperfused, it is probably a bleb- or bulla-containing portion of lung tissue.

INTRADERMAL TESTS.   The most frequently performed is the tuberculin test; a liquid containing the antigen is injected under the skin. If a red wheal forms at the site of injection 24 to 48 hours later, the patient has a present or past infection with tuberculosis.

FIGURE 3–17. Selective pulmonary angiography with multiple projections. Angiograms in the anteroposterior projection following injection of dye into the main pulmonary artery were normal. In contrast, angiograms after selective injections into the left main pulmonary artery in the oblique projection (*A*) reveal *possible* intraluminal filling defect (arrow); repeat study in lateral projection (*B*) reveals *obvious* large embolus (arrows). (From Hinshaw HC, Murray JF: *Diseases of the Chest*. 4th ed. Philadelphia, WB Saunders Company, 1980, p 48.)

BRONCHOSCOPY. The bronchoscope, a rigid tubular instrument, can be inserted through the mouth and the trachea, making examination of the bronchi possible as far as the segmental orifices. A flexible fiberoptic bronchoscope can be inserted considerably farther and can be used to obtain a biopsy of even peripheral lung lesions for definitive diagnosis. In addition, the flexible bronchoscope can be used to obtain pieces of lung tissue from patients with diffuse pulmonary disease (transbronchial biopsy) and to remove secretions, or mucous plugs. Bronchoscopy is most often performed when carcinoma is suspected, but it is also used to diagnose an inhaled foreign body as well as other conditions.

BRONCHOGRAPHY. In this radiographic technique used to visualize the trachea and bronchi, the bronchial tree is anesthetized with a topical anesthetic, then coated with an oily contrast medium. Bronchography is of value mainly for documenting the presence and extent of bronchiectasis (Fig. 3–20).

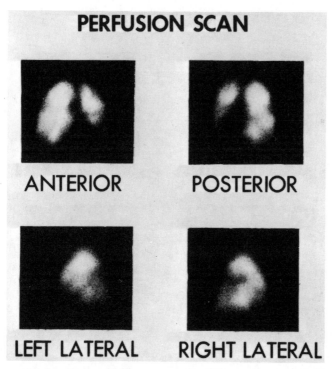

PERFUSION SCAN

ANTERIOR   POSTERIOR

LEFT LATERAL   RIGHT LATERAL

FIGURE 3–18.   Perfusion scintiscans. Perfusion lung scan with ^{99m}Tc-albumin of a 49-year-old man, who had been in a long leg cast for two weeks and who was complaining of chest pain and dyspnea, showing multiple segmental defects in all four views. Angiography confirmed presence of multiple pulmonary emboli.   (From Hinshaw HC, Murray JF: *Diseases of the Chest.* 4th ed. Philadelphia, WB Saunders Company, 1980, p 663.)

MEDIASTINOSCOPY.   During this examination, a rigid tube is inserted into the mediastinum from just above the sternal notch, and any lymph nodes visible can undergo biopsy. This technique is of special value in determining if lung cancer has spread to the mediastinal lymph nodes or if a mediastinal density represents metastatic spread.

PLEURAL ASPIRATION AND BIOPSY.   Once the presence of pleural fluid has been documented, a needle may be inserted into the chest to withdraw a sample for laboratory examination. Pleural biopsy is especially helpful if bacteriologic or pathologic examination reveals the presence of tubercle bacilli or malignant cells.

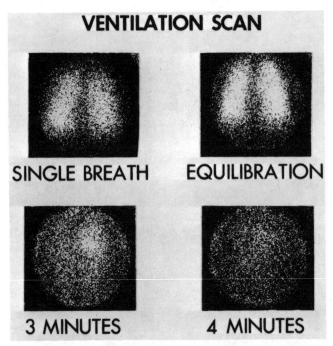

FIGURE 3–19.   Ventilation scintiscans. Ventilation lung scan with ^{133}Xe of the same patient described in Figure 3–18, showing even distribution of a single breath of the isotope, uniform labeling of both lungs at equilibration, and nearly even washout at three and four minutes. (There is slight retention in the right upper lung field.)   (From Hinshaw HC, Murray JF: *Diseases of the Chest.* 4th ed. Philadelphia, WB Saunders Company, 1980, p 664.)

OXYGEN TENSION (PaO$_2$), CARBON DIOXIDE TENSION (PaCO$_2$), AND pH.   These are determined by drawing an arterial blood sample from the radial artery in the wrist, the brachial artery above the elbow, or the femoral artery in the groin. If pulmonary function is poor, arterial oxygen tension is diminished, but carbon dioxide tension may be increased. The pH is diminished as well, indicating that the blood is abnormally acidic, a result of increased hydrogen ion concentration. This condition is referred to as respiratory acidosis.

MAGNETIC RESONANCE IMAGING   uses a powerful magnet and a computer to create images of body structures. MRI images of the chest show greater contrast between lesions and blood vessels than do CT scans (Fig. 3–21).

FIGURE 3–20.   Bronchography. Chest roentgenogram and three views from subsequent bronchography of a 20-year-old man with chronic cough, intermittent hemoptysis, and foul-smelling sputum. Slight increase in right-sided markings (*A*) is shown to be caused by bronchiectasis of the right upper and middle lobes (*B*, *C*, and *D*).   (From Hinshaw HC, Murray JC: *Diseases of the Chest.* 4th ed. Philadelphia, WB Saunders Company, 1980, p 598.)

SUMMARY OF THE HISTORY AND PHYSICAL EXAMINATION

HISTORY

I. Chief complaint—Why has the patient come for medical help?

II. Family and social history

    A. History of tuberculosis?

    B. History of allergic disorder or asthma?

FIGURE 3–21.   Bronchogenic carcinoma involving left hilum. CT scan (*A*), transverse magnetic resonance image (*B*), and coronal (*C*) gated magnetic resonance image. CT scan shows mass (arrow) lateral to the pulmonary artery. MRI images demonstrate that mass is clearly separable from the pulmonary artery and does not extend into the mediastinum; (A) aortic arch, (B) bronchus, (P) pulmonary artery. (From Higgins CB: The thorax. In *Magnetic Resonance Imaging of the Body.* Higgins CB, Hricak H (eds). New York, Raven Press, 1987, p 199.)

      C. Environmental air pollution?

      D. Cigarette smoking (evaluated in pack-years = packs per day × number of years smoked)

III. Occupational history

      A. Exposure to industrial dusts—silica, asbestos?

      B. Exposure to pigeons, parrots, canaries or parakeets? Psittacosis may result

      C. Residence in California's San Joaquin Valley? Consider coccidioidomycosis; histoplasmosis in patients from eastern or midwestern United States

IV. History of previous illness

      A. Tuberculosis

      B. Pneumonia or "pleurisy"

      C. Chest injuries and operations

V. Pain

    A. Pulmonary pain—usually occurs when the parietal pleura, major airways, chest wall, diaphragm, or mediastinal structures are affected by pathologic processes

    B. Pleural pain—usually localized, aggravated by chest expansion, may not be distinguishable from pulmonary pain

    C. Pain of intercostal neuritis—superficial, related to coughing, sneezing, straining

    D. Muscular pain—look for local tenderness to palpation

    E. Costochondral pain—dull, gnawing, aching, little relationship to movement

    F. Cardiac pain—"crushing" pain beneath the sternum, radiating into the shoulders, arms, or neck

    G. Pericardial pain—similar to pleural pain, relieved by sitting up and leaning forward

    H. Aortic pain—especially of a dissecting aneurysm, described as substernal, deep, boring, agonizing, tearing

    I. Pulmonary embolus—chest pain associated with shortness of breath, rarely hemoptysis, cough

VI. Cough

    A. Suggests abnormality when persistent

    B. Two types of cough

        1. Productive—clears airways of secretions

        2. Nonproductive—irritative, serves no useful purpose ("dry cough")

    C. Type of sputum suggests pathologic process

        1. Foul smelling—lung abscess

        2. Abundant, frothy, saliva-like—bronchoalveolar carcinoma

        3. Voluminous, pink, frothy—pulmonary edema

        4. Rust-colored—pneumococcal pneumonia

        5. Copious, purulent, brought up with posture change—bronchiectasis

VII. Hemoptysis—coughing up blood

    A. Most patients with hemoptysis have bronchitis, but some may be seriously ill

    B. Blood from gastrointestinal tract (hematemesis) or nasopharynx may be confused with blood from the lung

VIII. Dyspnea—shortness of breath or difficulty breathing

    A. Ask circumstances—association with climbing two flights of steps or walking a half block?

    B. Dyspnea is occasionally psychogenic or emotional

IX. Hoarseness
  A. Usually an abnormality of vocal cords
  B. May be due to lung tumor or aortic aneurysm damage of recurrent laryngeal nerve
X. Wheeze—a musical sound described fully in chapter five

PHYSICAL EXAMINATION

I. Inspection—general
  A. Evaluate breathlessness, wheezing, sputum, cough
  B. Observe skin for cyanosis and pallor, eruptions, nodules, scars
  C. Look for neck vein distention
  D. Examine fingers for tobacco stains, fingers and toes for clubbing
  E. Evaluate anteroposterior diameter relative to lateral diameter of chest wall
  F. Look for pectus carinatum ("pigeon breast"), pectus excavatum ("funnel chest"), kyphosis (abnormally increased spine curvature), scoliosis (lateral spine curvature), kyphoscoliosis
  G. Observe tracheal position; it should be midline
II. Inspection—respiratory motions
  A. Note whether chest expansion is bilaterally symmetric
  B. Look for abnormal breathing
    1. Bradypnea—abnormally slow breathing
    2. Tachypnea—abnormally fast breathing
    3. Apnea—temporary cessation of respiration
    4. Hyperpnea—increase in depth of breathing ("air hunger")
    5. Periodic respiration—alternating hyperpnea and apnea
    6. Sighing respiration, deep breaths interrupting normal rhythm, is commonly a sign of emotional tension
  C. Note mode of breathing—thoracic or abdominal
III. Palpation
  A. Examine neck, axillae, and supraclavicular fossae for lymph nodes; biopsy of these may be the only practical means of diagnosing lung cancer
  B. Palpate trachea to detect any deviation from the midline, or deviation anteriorly
  C. Palpate chest wall while patient says "one, two, three" or

"ninety-nine" to detect increased or decreased vibrations (vocal or tactile fremitus)

  D. Gauge respiratory motions of the rib margins to assess relative movement of the two sides of the chest

IV. Percussion—tapping body structures to produce a sound

  A. Percussion sounds from similar areas on each side of the chest should be compared

  B. Percuss to determine whether diaphragmatic motion is normal

V. Auscultation—see Chapter 4

BIBLIOGRAPHY

BATES BA: *A Guide to Physical Examination*. Philadelphia, JB Lippincott Company, 1974.

BOHADANA AB, PATEL R, KRAMAN SS: Contour maps of auscultatory percussion in healthy subjects and patients with large intrapulmonary lesions. *Lung* 167:359–372, 1989.

CONLAN AA, HURWITZ SS, KRIEGE L, NICOLAOU N, POOL R: Massive hemoptysis. Review of 123 cases. *J Thorac Cardiovasc Surg* 85:120–124, 1983.

DELP MH, MANNING RT: *Major's Physical Diagnosis*. Philadelphia, WB Saunders Company, 1980.

FORGACS P: *Lung Sounds*. London, Bailliere Tindall, 1978.

GONG H, SALVATIERRA C: Clinical efficacy of early and delayed fiberoptic bronchoscopy in patients with hemoptysis. *Am Rev Respir Dis* 124:221–225, 1981.

GRANT I: The respiratory system. In *Clinical Examination*. Macleod J (ed). Edinburgh, Churchill Livingstone, 1979.

HIGGINS CB: The thorax. In *Magnetic Resonance Imaging of the Body*. Higgins CB, Hricak HH (eds). New York, Raven Press, 1987.

HINSHAW HC, MURRAY JF: *Diseases of the Chest*. 4th ed. Philadelphia, WB Saunders Company, 1980.

IRWIN RS, CORRAO WM, PRATTER MR: Chronic persistent cough in the adult: The spectrum and frequency of causes and successful outcome of specific therapy. *Am Rev Respir Dis* 123:413–417, 1981.

KERSTEN L: *Comprehensive Respiratory Care. An Assessment Approach*. Philadelphia, WB Saunders Company, in preparation.

MURRAY JF: Diagnostic evaluation. History and physical examination. In *Textbook of Respiratory Medicine*. Murray JF, Nadel JA (eds). Philadelphia, WB Saunders Company, 1988, pp 431–451.

NAIDICH D, ZERHOUNI EA, SIEGELMAN SS. *Computed Tomography of the Thorax*. New York, Raven Press, 1984.

POE RH, ISRAEL RH, UTELL MJ, HALL WJ: Chronic cough: Bronchoscopy or pulmonary function testing? *Am Rev Respir Dis* 126:160–162, 1982.

PRIOR JA, SILBERSTEIN JS: *Physical Diagnosis*. 6th ed. St Louis, CV Mosby Company, 1981.

RABIN C: New or neglected signs in the diagnosis of chest disease. In *Pulmonary Diseases and Disorders*. Fishman AP (ed). New York, McGraw-Hill Book Company, 1980.

THROPE CW, FRIGHT WR, TOOP LJ, DAWSON KP: A microcomputer-based interactive cough sound analysis system. *Comput Methods Programs Biomed* 36(1):33–43, 1991.

4

NORMAL BREATH SOUNDS

How are the normal sounds of breathing produced? This question has puzzled investigators since the beginning of the nineteenth century. Researchers now believe that these normal sounds are produced by the turbulent flow of air in the lobar and segmental bronchi. No sounds are produced by air moving in and out of the alveoli, as the air flow here is slower and probably nonturbulent.

This chapter will discuss normal breath sounds by presenting these topics:

1. Auscultation.

2. Early experiments. One erroneously led to the conclusion that normal breath sounds are produced in the alveoli.

3. Turbulence and breath sounds. Rapidly flowing air moves in a noisy, turbulent manner; slowly flowing air moves in a silent, laminar manner. Because air flow is most turbulent in the trachea and first few generations of bronchi, normal breath sounds are most likely produced here.

4. Regional air flow and breath sounds. Studies of the lung have shown that there are regional differences in sound intensity at the apex and base of the lung. These fluctuations reflect differences that have been measured in regional air flow.

5. Variation of breath sounds with the heartbeat. Breath sounds over the left lower lobe of the lung become louder when the heart contracts and the adjacent lung tissue expands, lowering alveolar pressure and facilitating air flow into the left lower lobe. This observation again confirms the relationship of air flow to production of breath sounds.

67

6. Breath sounds at the mouth.
7. Breath sounds over the chest and trachea.
8. **Phonopneumography.** This technique allows the visual display of breath sounds. It has been used both for teaching and for breath sounds research, showing, for example, that the loudest point on the chest wall is the area immediately below the clavicle, anteriorly.

The field of breath sounds research has expanded greatly in the last few years; much of the recent work is described in this chapter, and it will provide background and understanding for anyone who wishes to follow new developments as they occur.

AUSCULTATION

With the patient sitting upright, comparative auscultation of the region overlying each pulmonary segment should be made. The stethoscope should be moved back and forth between comparable pulmonary segments on either side of the chest (Fig. 4–1). Auscultation should not be performed by moving the stethoscope down one side, then down the other. Each region should be listened to carefully while the patient is breathing through the mouth at a slightly increased rate and depth.

The examiner should first concentrate on inspiration—its length and its normal and adventitial components (crackles, wheezes, and so on; see Chapter 5). The examiner should then note the same phenomena in expiration.

The chest should always be auscultated in a quiet room. Radios and television sets should be turned off. The examiner should try to avoid listening over chest hair. When the hair moves against the diaphragm of the stethoscope during breathing, a crackling sound is produced that is quite similar to that heard within the lungs in certain pathologic conditions; when unavoidable, wetting the hair will reduce or prevent this phenomenon. The stethoscope should not be used over clothing, because the breath sounds will then be difficult to hear. The tubing should not touch clothing, bedsheets, or other objects, because artifactual noise will be produced. Four types of breath sounds are heard over the normal chest (Figs. 4–2 and 4–3):

1. *Normal vesicular.* This is a relatively soft, low-pitched sound, sometimes described as a sighing or gentle rustling; it is heard over most of the peripheral parts of the lung. The inspiratory phase is markedly longer than the expiratory phase, the I:E ratio being about 3:1. Expiration is much quieter than inspiration, usually being almost inaudible. There is no pause between inspiration and expiration.

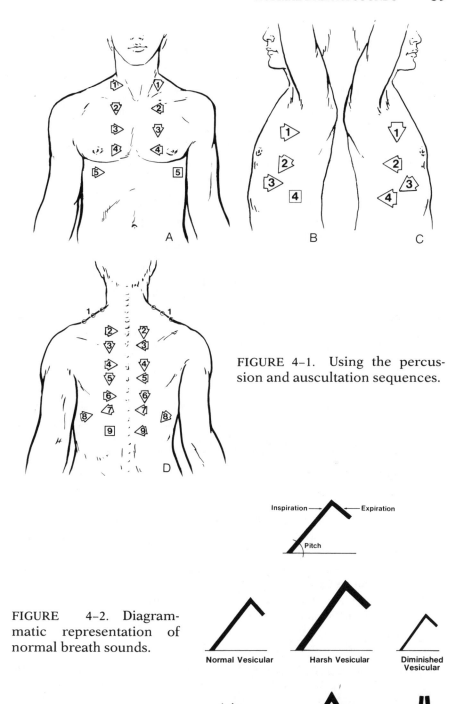

FIGURE 4–1. Using the percussion and auscultation sequences.

FIGURE 4–2. Diagrammatic representation of normal breath sounds.

Inspiration → ← Expiration

Pitch

Normal Vesicular

Harsh Vesicular

Diminished Vesicular

Bronchial

Bronchovesicular

Tracheal

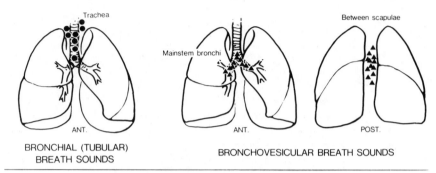

FIGURE 4–3.   Breath sounds over the normal chest.

The term *vesicular* is a misnomer. As will be discussed more fully later, the term came from experiments performed in the nineteenth century suggesting that the normal sounds arose in the alveoli, then called "vesicles." In fact, modern engineering concepts make it more likely that these sounds emanate from the turbulent flow of air in the lobar and segmental bronchi, not the alveoli.

2. *Bronchial.* These characteristically loud, high-pitched sounds resemble the sound of air blowing through a hollow pipe. Their expiratory phase is louder and longer than their inspiratory phase. They are normally present only over the manubrium, and a distinct pause can be heard between the inspiratory and expiratory phases. The appearance of bronchial sounds over the periphery of the lung may mean abnormal sound transmission because of consolidated lung tissue, as in pneumonia or atelectasis. This phenomenon will be dealt with in Chapter 5.

3. *Bronchovesicular.* These sounds are a mixture of bronchial and vesicular sounds. Their inspiratory and expiratory phases are about equal in length (I:E ratio = 1:1). They are normally audible in two places: (1) anteriorly, near the mainstem bronchi in the first and second intercostal spaces, and (2) posteriorly, between

TABLE 4–1. Physical Findings in Some Common Pulmonary Disorders.*

Disorder	Inspection	Palpation	Percussion	Auscultation
Bronchial asthma (acute attack)	Hyperinflation Use of accessory muscles	Impaired expansion Decreased fremitus	Hyperresonance Low diaphragms	Prolonged expiration Wheezes
Pneumothorax (complete)	Lag on affected side	Absent fremitus	Hyperresonant or tympanitic	Absent breath sounds
Pleural effusion (large)	Lag on affected side	Decreased fremitus Trachea and heart shifted away from affected side	Dullness or flatness	Absent breath sounds
Atelectasis (lobar obstruction)	Lag on affected side	Decreased fremitus Trachea and heart shifted toward affected side	Dullness or flatness	Absent breath sounds
Consolidation (pneumonia)	Possible lag or splinting on affected side	Increased fremitus	Dullness	Bronchial breath sounds Bronchophony Pectoriloquy

*From Hinshaw HC, Murray JF: *Diseases of the Chest.* 4th ed. Philadelphia, WB Saunders Company, 1980, p 23. Used by permission.

the scapulae. To hear them elsewhere may mean lung consolidation or other abnormality.

4. *Tracheal.* These sounds, not usually auscultated, are present over the extrathoracic portion of the trachea. They are very loud, are very high pitched, and have a hollow or harsh quality. The expiratory phase is slightly longer than the inspiratory phase.

I:E ratios of tracheal and bronchial sounds are about the same. The major determinant of the length of the expiratory sound is its loudness. At the lung bases, only the loudest portion of the sound can be heard; therefore, it seems short.

Physical findings in some common pulmonary disorders are presented in Table 4–1.

EARLY EXPERIMENTS

In 1819, René Théophile Laennec recorded the first description of the normal lung sound: "A slight but extremely distinct murmur answering to the entrance of air into and its expulsion from the air cells of the lung." At the time, no one was certain whether this sound was produced within the larynx or within the lungs themselves (Laennec, 1935; Murphy, 1981).

In 1884, J. F. Bullar, an English surgeon, made the first effort to elucidate the correct mechanism (Bullar, 1884). He constructed an artificial thorax made of an airtight, fluid-filled chamber with glass

FIGURE 4–4. In 1884, J. F. Bullar, an English surgeon, used this artificial thorax to investigate the origin of breath sounds. (From Bullar JF: Experiments to determine the origin of the respiratory sounds. *Proc R Soc Lond* 37:411–423, 1884.)

sides, which could be expanded and contracted with a bellows (Fig. 4–4). Within the artificial thorax he placed one of two sheep lungs, connected to the other (which was left outside) by its trachea and bronchi. Even when the trachea was plugged, he found that he could produce normal breath sounds. Bullar concluded correctly that these normal sounds were produced within the lungs but incorrectly surmised that they were generated as air passed from the terminal bronchioles into the alveoli. Years later, an American investigator, R. R. Hannon, performed other experiments confirming Bullar's observation that some normal sounds are produced in the lung (Hannon and Lyman, 1929).

TURBULENCE AND BREATH SOUNDS

Turbulence in the airstream is believed to be the source of normal breath sounds (Forgacs, 1978). To appreciate this fact fully, one should have some knowledge of the three types of fluid flow: (1) laminar flow, (2) turbulent flow, and (3) vortices.

LAMINAR FLOW. When a fluid, such as air, is flowing slowly along a straight, smooth pipe, it flows in streamlines or layers parallel with the walls of the pipe. The pressure driving the fluid is gradually dissipated by forces that occur between neighboring streamlines and between the gas and the walls of the pipe. Because there are no sudden changes or oscillations of pressure, no sound waves are generated.

TURBULENT FLOW. When the fluid flow reaches a critical velocity, the orderly arrangement of the streamlines breaks up, and small packets of gas begin to move at random across or against the general direction of flow. A common example of laminar and turbulent flow is the stream of smoke emanating from a lit cigarette (Fig. 4–5). Close to the cigarette, the flow is laminar, that is, smooth and regular. Farther away, the flow becomes more disorderly, that is, turbulent.

In turbulent flow, energy is transferred between colliding packets of gas, and transient pressure variations occur, generating sound. The noise produced by these rapid gas fluctuations varies at random in amplitude, with an even frequency distribution between 200 and 2000 Hz, or approximately the frequencies of normal speech. By analogy with the frequency spectrum of white light, such sound is often described as *white noise*.

Turbulence begins at a critical flow velocity. From experimental observations of gas flow and by calculation, investigators have learned that air flow is turbulent in the trachea and the first few generations of bronchi. In the peripheral bronchi, the slower flow becomes laminar and silent. Between these two regions an intermediate zone exists, extending from the segmental bronchi to the fifteenth generation of the airways. Here the laminar flow pattern is disrupted by vortices.

VORTICES. When a stream of gas emerges from a slit or circular orifice into a wider channel, the forces arising at the boundary between the stream and the surrounding fluid generate whirlpools, or

FIGURE 4–5. Turbulent flow and laminar flow. When the flow of a fluid reaches a critical velocity, the orderly arrangement of the streamlines breaks up, and small packets of gas begin to move at random across or against the general direction of flow. A common example of laminar and turbulent flow is the smoke stream emanating from a lit cigarette. Close to the cigarette the flow is laminar, that is, smooth and regular. Farther away, the flow becomes more disorderly, that is, turbulent.

FIGURE 4–6.   Vortices. When a stream of gas emerges from a slit or circular orifice into a wider channel, the forces arising at the boundary between the stream and the surrounding fluid generate whirlpools or vortices.

vortices. Vortices are also produced when a curvature or angle in the pipe forces flow to change direction abruptly. These conditions cause the gas stream to separate into layers that move forward at different velocities. The slower streams are turned into circular motion by the force of the high-velocity streams flowing alongside (Fig. 4–6). The resulting noise has a wide frequency spectrum, the lower frequencies probably being more prominent in the periphery of the lung.

Two observations support the view that high air flow rate, vortices, and turbulence produce breath sounds in the larger airways: (1) the relationship between regional air flow rate and breath sounds; and (2) the variation with the heartbeat of the breath sounds over the left lower lobe of the lung.

REGIONAL AIR FLOW AND BREATH SOUNDS

Measurements of inspiratory breath sounds through the chest wall show that there are regional differences in sound intensity at the apex and base of the lung (Leblanc et al., 1970; Ploysongsang et al., 1977; Shykoff et al, 1988).

In a normal individual in the upright position, breath sounds at the apex become progressively fainter during inspiration from residual volume. In contrast, at the base, the breath sounds are relatively faint at the beginning of inspiration; their intensity increases to a maximum at 50 percent of the vital capacity (Fig. 4–7). These fluctuations reflect differences that have been measured in regional air flow rates. In the

FIGURE 4–7. Relative intensity of breath sounds plotted against lung volume (as percentage of vital capacity) in one subject. Note that the breath sounds at the apex become progressively fainter during inspiration. In contrast, at the base, the breath sounds are relatively faint at the beginning of inspiration; their intensity increases to a maximum at 50 percent of the vital capacity. These results correlated well with the differences in regional distribution of ventilation found with radioactive gases. (From Leblanc P, Macklem PT, Ross WRD: Breath sounds and distribution of pulmonary ventilation. *Am Rev Respir Dis* 102:10–16, 1970.)

apex, air flow begins immediately, regardless of the initial lung volume. At the base, the inspiratory air flow does not begin until the dependent airways, which are normally closed at low lung volumes, reopen.

VARIATION OF BREATH SOUNDS WITH HEARTBEAT

In some healthy individuals, breath sounds over the left lower lobe rise and fall in synchrony with the heartbeat. Usually, they are loudest during systole, when contraction of the ventricles allows the adjacent lung tissue to expand, lowering alveolar pressure and facilitating gas flow into the left lower lobe. Simultaneous recordings of the electrocardiogram and the breath sounds over the left lower lobe verify that the sounds become more intense at the R wave and reach their peak at the

FIGURE 4–8. Variations of breath sounds with heartbeat. In some healthy individuals, breath sounds over the left lower lobe rise and fall in synchrony with the heartbeat. Usually, they are loudest during systole, when contraction of the ventricles allows the adjacent lung tissue to expand, lowering gas pressure and facilitating gas flow into the left lower lobe. Simultaneous recordings of the electrocardiogram and the breath sounds over the left lower lobe verify that the sounds become more intense at the R wave and reach their peak at the T wave.   (From Forgacs P: *Lung Sounds.* London, Baillière Tindall, 1978.)

T wave (Fig. 4–8). This peak may be as much as 40 percent above the mean. It is interesting to note that in some people an opposite effect is associated with the heartbeat: the breath sounds become quieter during ventricular systole. Apparently, the movement of the heart into the left lower lobe has compressed the lung and transiently reduced the regional air flow rate.

BREATH SOUNDS AT THE MOUTH

Why are sounds at the mouth different from sounds heard through the chest wall? Apparently because of the different paths of transmission. In large tubes, such as the trachea and main bronchi, sound travels well and reaches the mouth almost unfiltered. However, sounds that must travel through the lung and chest wall are filtered; they fall into a relatively narrow range of low frequencies, with a steep fall in amplitude above 200 Hz. In contrast, the breath sounds at the mouth consist of a broad range of evenly distributed frequencies between 200 and 2000 cycles (Fig. 4–9). In other words, the chest wall and lung are acting as a so-called low pass filter and are allowing only the low frequencies to pass through.

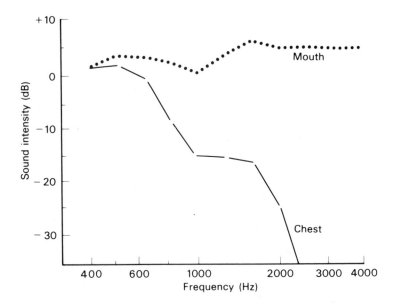

FIGURE 4–9. Intensity and frequency of breath sounds transmitted through the mouth and the chest. Note that the sounds traveling through the chest wall and lung are filtered, falling into a relatively narrow range of low frequencies with a steep fall in amplitude above 200 Hz. In contrast, the breath sounds at the mouth consist of a broad range of evenly distributed frequencies between 200 and 2000 Hz. (From Forgacs P: *Lung Sounds*. London, Baillière Tindall, 1978.)

Breath Sounds Over the Chest and Trachea

Breath sounds transmitted through the chest fade out during expiration, whereas those over the trachea can be heard throughout the respiratory cycle. There are at least two reasons for this:

1. Although rate of air flow falls continuously during expiration, the breath sounds over the trachea are so loud that they remain above the threshold of hearing throughout the respiratory cycle. The sounds transmitted through the chest wall are much fainter, and they contain mostly low frequencies, to which the ear is less sensitive. Thus, the breath sounds become too soft to hear early in expiration.

2. During inspiration, turbulence is most likely generated and carried farther toward the periphery of the lung than during expiration. Because the turbulence moves away from the chest wall during expiration, the resulting faint breath sounds are absorbed by the lung before they reach the stethoscope.

BREATH SOUNDS IN CHILDREN

Clinicians who auscultate the chests of normal children note that the sound quality varies with age. In fact, studies of the amplitude–frequency spectrum of the sounds confirms that there is a change with age of the frequency content. The breath sounds of very young children have more high-frequency components than do those of adults; therefore, they sound higher pitched (Hidalgo et al., 1991; Kanga and Kraman, 1986).

PHONOPNEUMOGRAPHY

Phonopneumograms, which are visual displays of breath sounds, are used both as an analytic research device and as a clinical teaching tool. They are useful research tools because a visual plot of a breath sound can be analyzed in considerably more detail than can the same sound heard through a stethoscope. As a teaching device, phonopneumograms can present slowly and clearly to the eye a sound pattern that might, to the ear, be transient and difficult to interpret.

Some of the most useful early phonopneumograms were recorded by Dr. Victor A. McKusick in 1955 (Figs. 4–10 and 4–11). McKusick used a special device called a sound spectrograph and made the first detailed frequency analysis of the sounds. He showed, for example, that the normal inspiratory vesicular sounds were of maximal intensity at a frequency of about 200 Hz and decreased rapidly thereafter (McKusick et al., 1955). He found no sound energy at more than 500 Hz. As was pointed out in Chapter 2, the ear is relatively insensitive to sounds in this frequency range; thus, breath sounds are more difficult to perceive accurately than is normal speech.

In 1972, Weiss and Carlson published calibrated amplitude plots of breath sounds that were recorded on tape and then fed into an oscilloscope (Weiss and Carlson, 1972). These plots revealed the overall amplitude of the sounds during inspiration and expiration (Fig. 4–12).

In 1971, Dr. David. W. Cugell, of the Northwestern University School of Medicine, pointed out the importance of both phonopneumograms and breath sound recordings in teaching chest auscultation to medical students (Cugell, 1971). He prepared a questionnaire to determine the level of interest in tape recordings of breath sounds, and found that although considerable interest existed, little use was made of audio-visual materials. The dearth of such material at the time prompted Dr. Cugell to test and describe an admirable system for making phonopneumograms and breath sound recordings.

The phonopneumogram is especially useful if it is displayed with a plotted graph that simultaneously shows the precise phase of inspi-

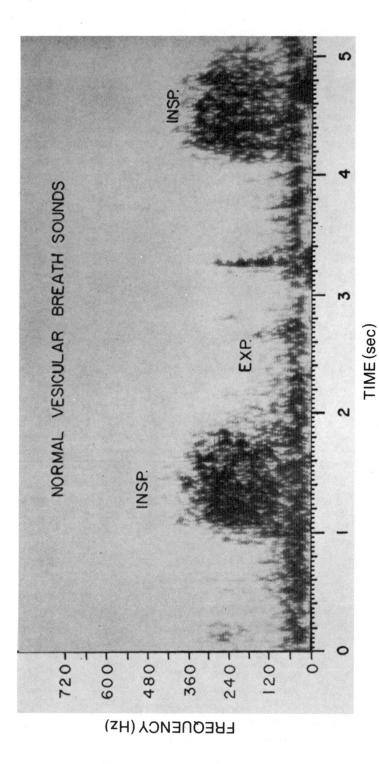

FIGURE 4-10. Sound spectrogram of normal vesicular breath sounds made by Dr. Victor McKusick in 1955. The intensity of the sounds is represented by the darkness of the patterns in the tracing. Note that inspiration is louder and higher pitched than expiration.   (From McKusick VA, Jenkins WT, Webb GN: The acoustic basis of the chest examination: Studies by means of sound spectrography. *Am Rev Tuberc* 72:12–34, 1955.)

FIGURE 4-11. Tracheal breath sounds recorded by Dr. Victor McKusick on the sound spectrograph. Note that inspiration and expiration are about the same pitch. (From McKusick VA, Jenkins WT, Webb GN: The acoustic basis of the chest examination: Studies by means of sound spectrography. *Am Rev Tuberc* 72:12–34, 1955.)

FIGURE 4-12. Calibrated amplitude plots of breath sounds displayed on the screen of an oscilloscope. Note that in #1, which was recorded over the trachea (bronchial breathing), expiration (E) is louder and longer than inspiration (I). In #2, which was recorded over the middle lobe (bronchovesicular breathing), intensity of expiration is markedly reduced. In #3, which was recorded at the lung base (vesicular breathing), inspiration is again louder and longer than expiration. (From Weiss EB, Carlson CJ: Recording of breath sounds. *Am Rev Respir Dis* 105:835–839, 1972.)

ration or expiration (Banaszak et al., 1973). This double display is accomplished by adding a device called a pneumotachometer to create the phase chart and display the velocity of breathing. The apparatus for making the entire recording is shown in Figure 4–13, and a typical recording is shown in Figure 4–14.

A drawback to the phonopneumogram just presented is that normal lung sounds cannot be visually distinguished from abnormal or adventitious sounds, such as crackles and wheezes. Their frequency is simply too high. To circumvent this problem, Dr. Raymond L. Murphy,

RECORDING SYSTEM

DATA ANALYSIS SYSTEM

FIGURE 4–13. System for simultaneous recording of breath sounds and breathing velocity. CRO = cathode ray oscilloscope. (From Banaszak EF, Kory RC, Snider GL: Phonopneumography. *Am Rev Respir Dis* 107:449–455, 1973.)

FIGURE 4–14. Typical recording made with the system shown in Figure 4–13. The system is set up to be most sensitive to sounds at 100 Hz. Sound intensity is represented by the upper tracing, flow rate by the lower tracing. (From Banaszak EF, Kory RC, Snider GL: Phonopneumography. *Am Rev Respir Dis* 107:449–455, 1973.)

CONVENTIONAL (100 mm/sec)   EXPANDED (800 mm/sec)

(a) NORMAL VESICULAR INSPIRATORY SOUND

(b) INSPIRATORY RALES AT POSTERIOR LUNG BASE

(c) SONOROUS RHONCHUS

(d) SIBILANT RHONCHUS (Wheeze)

(e) NORMAL TRACHEAL INSPIRATION

FIGURE 4-15. Amplitude versus time plots of typical lung sounds, showing that the expanded time scales in the right column reveal visually distinct patterns that are not well seen in conventional plots. Time is on the horizontal axis and amplitude is on the vertical axis. The effective chart recorder speeds are 100 mm per second and 800 mm per second. (From Murphy RLH, Holford SK, Knowler WC: Visual lung sound characterization by time-expanded wave form analysis. *N Engl J Med* 296:968–971, 1977.)

Jr. used a technique known as time-expanded wave form analysis (Murphy et al., 1977). After storing the recorded sounds in the memory of a computer, he replayed the signal at a much slower rate. These time-expanded wave forms of typical sounds showed patterns that allowed the various categories of sound to be visually distinguished from one another (Fig. 4–15). In addition, artifactual sounds could be distinguished from true lung sounds (Fig. 4–16).

Dr. Steve S. Kraman has made innovative use of phonopneumography. Dr. Kraman has employed a technique, subtraction phonopneumography, to determine the site of production of respiratory sounds (Kraman, 1980).

In subtraction phonopneumography, simultaneous recordings of the lung sounds are made from two different areas of the chest. These recordings are then analyzed to determine whether they represent (1) the same or a similar sound transmitted to each microphone from one or more distant sources, or (2) dissimilar sounds transmitted from

(a) VOICE

(b) 1st HEART SOUND

(c) HAIR NOISE

(d) SKIN NOISE

FIGURE 4-16. Artifactual sounds displayed as time-expanded wave forms have different patterns from the lung sounds shown in Figure 4-15. Voice sounds recorded with the microphone on the subject's chest are shown in (A); the first heart sound recorded on the left anterior part of the chest is shown in (B); vesicular sounds with superimposed noise of the microphone moving over chest hair is shown in (C); and a plot resulting from sliding the microphone across the skin is shown in (D). (From Murphy RLH, Holford SK, Knowler WC: Visual lung sound characterization by time-expanded wave form analysis. *N Engl J Med* 296:968–971, 1977.)

sources located near each microphone. Because the normal sounds of breathing are well heard over virtually all of the chest surface, one may assume that a single, centrally produced sound would be transmitted through the lung to the periphery and would arrive in an identical form (in phase) at two different locations on the chest wall that are equidistant from the source. However, a peripherally produced sound, that is, a sound emanating from the subpleural alveolar sacs, would sound loudest to the microphone under which it was produced and would be different from a peripherally produced sound generated directly under the second microphone; in other words, the two sounds would be dissimilar in phase. Thus, if one sound is electronically subtracted from another, two similar sounds in phase will cancel each other out, whereas two dissimilar sounds will not.

During this experiment, Dr. Kraman found that when the microphones were placed 4 cm apart, normal people had at least 50 percent cancellation of the normal inspiratory sound. In contrast, in recordings of pleural friction rubs, there was no cancellation with microphones placed over opposite lungs. As a result, he concluded that the source of the main component of the normal inspiratory sound is more peripheral than the mainstem bronchi but farther from the chest wall than the pleura; how far is impossible to tell.

Dr. Kraman found that expiratory sounds come from a more central location than inspiratory sounds. In fact, some of the sound seemed to be emanating from above the point—the carina—where the trachea bifurcates into the two mainstem bronchi. Because students are commonly taught that sounds from the larynx are transmitted to the periphery and form part of the normal vesicular breath sounds (Bushnell,

1921), Dr. Kraman designed a second experiment to test the validity of this notion (Kraman, 1981).

The study was designed around the hypothesis that if the laryngeal noise forms an audible part of the vesicular sound heard on the chest wall during quiet breathing, then the vesicular sound should get louder during voluntarily produced noisy breathing. However, no such thing happened. Sounds were recorded from the larynx and four sites on the chest wall simultaneously during quiet breathing and during voluntarily produced noisy breathing. Despite severalfold increases in the amplitude of the laryngeal noise in both inspiration and expiration, the amplitude of the simultaneously recorded vesicular sound correlated only with flow rates and was completely unaffected by changes in laryngeal sound amplitude (Fig. 4–17). Therefore, during quiet breathing in

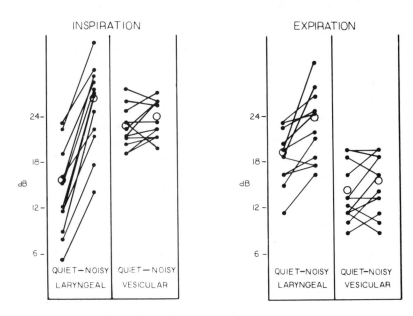

FIGURE 4–17. Relative amplitude of quiet and noisy breaths recorded from the larynx and four positions on the chest wall. The closed circles represent the intensity of each breath. The open circles represent the mean intensity of 12 breaths. Note that over the larynx during inspiration, the noisy breaths are significantly louder than the quiet breaths, whereas over the chest wall (vesicular) there is no significant difference between the amplitudes of the quiet and noisy breaths. The situation is similar in expiration. These findings demonstrate that during quiet breathing in healthy subjects, no detectable laryngeal noise can be heard in the vesicular breath sounds. (From Kraman S: Does laryngeal noise contribute to the vesicular lung sound? *Am Rev Respir Dis* 124:292–294, 1981.)

healthy subjects, no detectable component of the laryngeal noise is likely to reach the periphery.

Dr. Dennis O'Donnell and Dr. Kraman, using automated phono-pneumography, have also attempted to document the relative intensity patterns of lung sounds on the chest wall. By employing computerized analysis, they were able to record more than 50 positions on each side of the chest wall in eight normal subjects within a relatively short time. They found that, in general, the loudest point on the chest wall is the area immediately below the clavicle, anteriorly. Furthermore, chest wall thickness is not a major determinant of the amplitude of the vesicular sounds recorded on the surface of the chest. These sounds are distributed in an irregular succession of sound hills and valleys, with the loudest areas at the apices and bases (Fig. 4–18). The right or left lung sound intensities, although proportional to air flow at any one site, may vary by a considerable degree when compared with equally ventilated corresponding areas over the opposite lung (O'Donnell and Kraman, 1982), although the sound intensity at the left apex is always louder

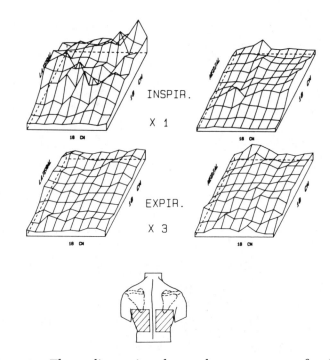

FIGURE 4–18.   Three-dimensional sound contour map of a single subject. Note that the sound is distributed in an irregular succession of hills and valleys over the chest wall.   (From Dosani R, Kraman SS: Lung sound intensity variability in normal men. A contour phonopneumographic study. *Chest* 83:628–631, 1983.)

than or equal to that at the right (Kraman, 1983) and is linearly associated with airflow (Kraman, 1984). The finding of sound hills and valleys is most surprising because many researchers had believed that lung sound intensity was relatively uniform over the chest of normal subjects (Dosani and Kraman, 1983).

Another application of phonopneumography, now in the experimental stages, is the monitoring of patients undergoing general anes-

VENTILATION OF TRACHEA   VENTILATION OF ESOPHAGUS

FIGURE 4–19. Lung sound patterns of patients undergoing anesthesia displayed on an oscilloscope screen. The pictures on the upper and lower left show that the endotracheal tube is properly placed, ventilating the trachea. The pictures on the upper and lower right show that the endotracheal tube has been improperly placed, and the esophagus is being ventilated.   (From Huang KC, Kraman SS, Wright BD: Video stethoscope: A simple method for assuring continuous bilateral lung ventilation during anesthesia.) (Reprinted with permission from the International Anesthesia Research Society from *Anesth Analg* 62:586–589, 1983.)

FIGURE 4–20.   Lung sound patterns resulting from ventilation of trachea (upper trace) and right mainstem bronchus (lower trace) in the same patient.   (From Huang KC, Kraman SS, Wright BD: Video stethoscope: A simple method for assuring continuous bilateral lung ventilation during anesthesia.) (Reprinted with permission from the International Anesthesia Research Society from *Anesth Analg* 62:586–589, 1983.)

thesia. Although mortality related to anesthesia is low, incorrect placement of the endotracheal tube during intubation is still a hazard. Huang, Kraman, and Wright developed a simple method of monitoring the ventilation of both lungs (Huang et al., 1983). They affixed a microphone to the skin overlying each side of the chest at a location at which preliminary auscultation showed that breath sounds could be heard. The sounds from each microphone were amplified and displayed on an oscilloscope screen in a so-called X–Y format. The patterns on the screen permitted easy verification of proper endotracheal tube placement, and improper placement of the tube in the right mainstem bronchus or the esophagus was readily detected (Figs. 4–19 and 4–20).

STUDY HELPS

1. Name and describe the four types of breath sounds heard over the normal chest.
2. Where are the normal vesicular breath sounds produced? What type of air flow causes these sounds?
3. Describe the regional differences in sound intensity at the apex and base of the lung.
4. What effect does contraction of the ventricles of the heart have on breath sounds heard over the left lower lobe?
5. Why are breath sounds that are heard at the mouth different from those that are heard through the chest wall?
6. Why do breath sounds that are heard over the chest fade out during expiration, while those over the trachea do not?
7. Does laryngeal noise transmitted to the chest wall form part of the normal vesicular breath sounds?

BIBLIOGRAPHY

AUSTRHEIM O, KRAMAN SS: The effect of low density gas breathing on vesicular lung sounds. *Respiration Physiology* 60:145–155, 1985.

BANASZAK EF, KORY RC, SNIDER GL: Phonopneumography. *Am Rev Respir Dis* 107:449–455, 1973.

BULLAR JF: Experiments to determine the origin of the respiratory sounds. *Proc R Soc Lond* 37:411–423, 1884.

BUSHNELL GE: The mode of production of the so-called vesicular murmur of respiration. *JAMA* 77:2104–2106, 1921.

CUGELL DW: Use of tape recordings of respiratory sound and breathing pattern for instruction in pulmonary auscultation. *Am Rev Respir Dis* 104:948–950, 1971.

DOSANI R, KRAMAN SS: Lung sound intensity variability in normal men. A contour phonopneumographic study. *Chest* 83:628–631, 1983.

FORGACS P: *Lung Sounds.* London, Baillière Tindall, 1978.

HANNON RR, LYMAN RS: Studies on pulmonary acoustics. II. The transmission of tracheal sounds through freshly exenterated sheep's lungs. *Am Rev Tuberc* 19:360–375, 1929.

HIDALGO HA, WEGMANN MJ, WARING WW: Frequency spectra of normal breath sounds in childhood. *Chest* 100(4):999–1002, 1991.

HUANG KC, KRAMAN SS, WRIGHT BD: Video stethoscope: A simple method for assuring continuous bilateral lung ventilation during anesthesia. *Anesth Analg* 62:586–589, 1983.

KANGA JF, KRAMAN SS: Comparison of the lung sounds frequency spectra of infants and adults. *Pediatr Pulmonol* 2:292–295, 1986.

KRAMAN SS: Determination of the site of production of respiratory sounds by subtraction phonopneumography. *Am Rev Respir Dis* 122:303–309, 1980.

KRAMAN SS: Does laryngeal noise contribute to the vesicular lung sound? *Am Rev Respir Dis* 124:292–294, 1981.

KRAMAN SS: Lung sounds: Relative sites of origin and comparative amplitudes in normal subjects. *Lung* 161:57–64, 1983.

KRAMAN SS: Speed of low frequency sound through the lungs of normal men. *J Appl Physiol: Resp Environ Exercise Physiol* 55(6):1862–1867, 1983.

KRAMAN SS: The relationship between airflow and lung sound amplitude in normal subjects. *Chest* 86(2):225–229, 1984.

KRAMAN SS: Effects of lung volume and airflow on the frequency spectrum of vesicular lung sounds. *Respiration Physiology* 66:1–9, 1986.

KRAMAN SS, AUSTRHEIM O: Comparison of lung sound and transmitted sound amplitude in normal men. *Clin Res* 31:418A, 1983.

LEBLANC P, MACKLEM PT, ROSS WRD: Breath sounds and distribution of pulmonary ventilation. *Am Rev Respir Dis* 102:10–16, 1970.

LAENNEC RTH: *A Treatise on the Diseases of the Chest and Mediate Auscultation.* Translated from the French by John Forbes. New York, Samuel Wood and Sons, 1935.

MARTINI P, MÜLLER H: Studien über das Bronchialatmen. *Dtsch Arch F Klin Med* 143:159–173, 1923.

MCKUSICK VA, JENKINS JT, WEBB GN: The acoustic basis of the chest examination: Studies by means of sound spectrography. *Am Rev Tuberc* 72:12–34, 1955.

MURPHY RLH: Auscultation of the lung: Past lessons, future possibilities. *Thorax* 36:99–107, 1981.

MURPHY RL, HOLFORD SK, KNOWLER WC: Visual lung sound characterization by time expanded wave form analysis. *N Engl J Med* 296:968–971, 1977.

NAIRN JR, TURNER-WARWICK M: Breath sounds in emphysema. *Br J Dis Chest* 63:29–37, 1969.

O'DONNELL DM, KRAMAN SS: Vesicular lung sound amplitude mapping by auto-mated flow-gated phonopneumography. *J Appl Physiol* 53:603–609, 1982.

PLOYSONGSANG Y, MARTIN RR, Ross WRD et al.: Breath sounds and regional ventilation. *Am Rev Respir Dis* 116:187–199, 1977.

PLOYSONGSANG Y, IYER VK, RAMAMOORTHY PA: Reproducibility of the vesicular breath sounds in normal subjects. *Respiration* 58(3–4): 158–162, 1991.

SHYKOFF BE, PLOYSONGSANG Y, CHANG HK: Airflow and normal lung sounds. *Am Rev Respir Dis* 137:872–876, 1988.

WEISS EB, CARLSON CJ: Recording of breath sounds. *Am Rev Respir Dis* 105:835, 939, 1972.

5

ABNORMAL BREATH SOUNDS

Many distinctive sounds are generated by a diseased lung. These may be roughly grouped into two broad categories: (1) adventitious (accidental) sounds—crackles, wheezes, pleural friction rubs; and (2) abnormally transmitted sounds—egophony, pectoriloquy, bronchophony, bronchial breathing, and abnormally diminished breath sounds. Recent scientific investigations, aided by advances in acoustics and electronics, provide insights into the mechanism of production of these sounds.

TERMINOLOGY: MAKING A CASE FOR CONSISTENCY

When Laennec first described adventitious lung sounds in the nineteenth century, he classified them as "rales" and then added adjectives for further clarification: crepitant (crackling), sibilant (high-pitched), sonorous (low-pitched). But "rale" had an unpleasant association with the rattle of the secretions in the airways of the dying; in order to spare the feelings of these patients, Laennec used the synonym "rhonchus" (Greek for snore) at the bedside (Robertson and Cope, 1957). Over the years, clinicians added many other adjectives, which, in fact, have no precise meaning and should not be used: wet rales, dry rales, sticky rales, bubbling rales, atelectatic rales, consonating rales (Cugell, 1978; Hudson et al., 1976). To confuse matters still more, "rhonchus" and "wheeze" came to be used interchangeably.

In 1975, the Joint Committee on Pulmonary Nomenclature of the American College of Chest Physicians–American Thoracic Society recategorized the two principal adventitious sounds: (1) "rale" for a discontinuous sound, also called a crackle; and (2) "rhonchus" for a continuous sound, which could also be called a wheeze.

In 1980, the American Thoracic Society further recategorized these sounds: (1) crackles (coarse and fine), (2) wheeze, and (3) rhonchus.

British investigators using acoustic criteria have modified the terminology for adventitious sounds still further by using only the terms crackle (coarse and fine) and wheeze (high-pitched and low-pitched). The British terms will be used in this chapter. The reader should be aware that in the pulmonary literature, a high-pitched wheeze may be called a sibilant rhonchus, whereas a low-pitched wheeze may be referred to as a sonorous rhonchus. Moreover, coarse crackles may be called low-pitched crackles and fine crackles may be called high-pitched crackles.

ADVENTITIOUS SOUNDS

Crackles

Crackles are short, explosive, nonmusical sounds. In addition to the coarse and fine classification mentioned previously, they may be described as to quantity (scanty or profuse) and timing (inspiratory or expiratory, early or late). They may be heard through the chest wall and sometimes at the mouth.

Laennec gave a very good qualitative description of the crackling sound; he compared it to the sound produced by heating salt in a frying pan. Modern time-expanded wave form analysis shows that the two sounds are indeed quite similar (Murphy, 1981).

In the past, crackles were attributed to bubbling secretions in the airways. This explanation is probably correct when the trachea and main bronchi are full of sputum and when the crackling is both inspiratory and expiratory. However, in other diseases, when there is no sputum, and when crackling is confined to inspiration, this explanation cannot be valid (Forgacs, 1978b).

The most widely accepted cause of crackling, described by Dr. Paul Forgacs, is the explosive equalization of gas pressure between two compartments of the lung, when a closed section of the airways separating them suddenly opens (Fig. 5–1). Several observations lend support to this notion.

In excised lungs, inflation is not accompanied by crackling unless the lung is deflated at the start of the experiment to the point at which some groups of alveoli under the pleura are seen to be airless. Under these circumstances, the lung does not inflate smoothly or evenly; instead, small groups of alveoli expand suddenly all over the surface.

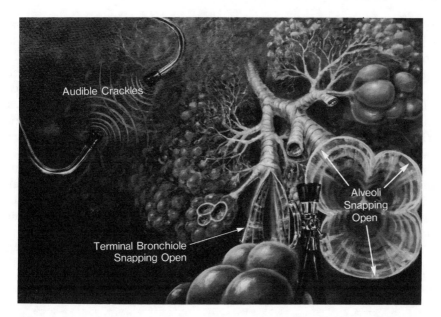

FIGURE 5–1.   The primary source of crackling is the explosive equalization of gas pressure between two compartments of the lung when a closed section of airway separating them suddenly opens.   (Illustration by Edward M. Jones.)

This random reinflation is accompanied by crackling, which stops as soon as the whole lung is re-aerated.

Another important clue to the genesis of crackling is the recurrent rhythm, characterized by similar spacing and relative loudness of successive crackles that can often be recognized in several consecutive respiratory cycles (Fig. 5–2). The recurrent rhythm indicates that the airways responsible for individual crackles open in the same sequence

FIGURE 5–2.   Simultaneous recording of inspiratory crackles and air flow rate shows a repetitive pattern of crackles (short vertical lines) in the two breaths.   (From Nath AR, Capel LH: Inspiratory crackles and mechanical events of breathing. *Thorax* 29:695–698, 1974.) (Reprinted by permission of the New England Journal of Medicine.)

and at approximately the same lung volume. Nath and Capel have confirmed that the reopening of each airway and, therefore, the timing of each crackle, are closely linked to the transpulmonary pressure; this was accomplished by simultaneous recording of sound amplitude and esophageal pressure, which is equivalent to pleural pressure (Nath and Capel, 1974b). In several consecutive respiratory cycles, crackles, identified by their spacing and relative amplitude, occurred at the same transpulmonary pressure (Fig. 5–3). The significance of the experiments described in this paragraph is that these crackles, because of their close relationship to transpulmonary pressure and their similarity in each respiratory cycle, must be due to the sudden opening of airways. They cannot be due to bubbling secretions in the airways; if they were, they would not be related to transpulmonary pressure and would not sound similar in each respiratory cycle.

In Japan, Mori has used the technique of time-expanded wave

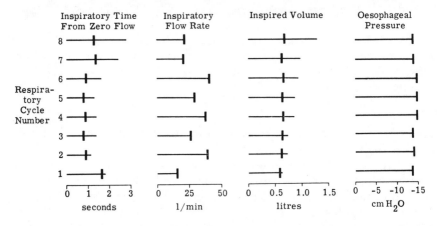

FIGURE 5–3. Results of experiment showing that reopening of each airway and timing of each crackle are closely linked to the transpulmonary pressure. From left to right, the length of the horizontal line represents the inspiratory time, the inspiratory flow rate, the inspired volume, and the transpulmonary pressure. The short vertical line represents the occurrence of a particular crackle, repeating through eight breaths. Note in the last two columns that the crackle occurred at a similar inspired volume and transpulmonary (esophageal) pressure, although the total inspired volume varied in the eight breaths. But the occurrence of this crackle is not closely related to the inspiratory time and inspiratory flow rate (first two columns). (From Nath AR, Capel LH: Inspiratory crackles and mechanical events of breathing. *Thorax* 29:695–698, 1974.) (Reprinted by permission of the New England Journal of Medicine.)

FIGURE 5-4. Amplitude versus time plots of lung sounds recorded from a patient with pulmonary tuberculosis and thoracoplasty during three consecutive respiratory cycles. Note the repetitive appearance of crackles with almost identical wave forms. The *starting segment* of the wave form (abcd) and the *decay segment* (1234) can also be seen. (From Mori M, Kinoshita M, Morinari H, et al.: Waveform and spectral analysis of crackles. *Thorax* 35:843–850, 1980.) (Reprinted by permission of the New England Journal of Medicine.)

form analysis to study crackles, elaborating on the work of Nath and Capel (Mori et al., 1980). Mori found that crackles occurred at the same point in the respiratory cycle and that repetitive crackles had identical wave forms (Fig. 5–4). Characteristically, the wave forms were separable into two segments, an initial "starting segment" and a subsequent "decay segment." The starting segment is apparently a shock wave caused by the abrupt opening of an airway. The subsequent decay segment is the result of the shock wave exciting a resonator in the lung. To test this shock wave-resonator hypothesis, Mori constructed a crackle simulator consisting of a syringe, a microphone, and a bottle resonator (Fig. 5–5) and was successful in obtaining wave forms similar to those of crackles.

Nath and Capel have shown that the timing of crackles in the inspiratory cycle can be used to distinguish the pulmonary diseases, which are discussed next (Nath and Capel, 1974a, 1980).

Crackles in Restrictive and Obstructive Disease

Early inspiratory crackles (Fig. 5–6) are characteristic of patients with severe airway obstruction. These crackles appear to be produced in the proximal and larger airways. They are frequently well transmitted to the mouth, are few in number, and are heard at one or both lung bases. An important feature of these crackles is that they are

FIGURE 5-5. Crackle simulator consisting of a syringe (1), a microphone (2), and a bottle (3), with its internal surface covered with polyurethane foam (4). The simulated crackles are produced by applying commercial paste to the orifice of the syringe and moving the piston up and down slowly. The vernier caliper at the bottom indicates 5 cm. The wave forms generated are similar to those of actual crackles. (From Mori M, Kinoshita K, Morinari H, et al.: Waveform and spectral analysis of crackles. *Thorax* 35:843–850, 1980.) (Reprinted by permission of the New England Journal of Medicine.)

FIGURE 5-6. Phonopneumogram of early inspiratory crackles (short vertical lines). Note that this is a simultaneous recording of both the crackles and the air flow rate. (From Nath AR, Capel LH: Inspiratory crackles—early and late. *Thorax* 29:223–227, 1974.) (Reprinted by permission of the New England Journal of Medicine.)

not silenced by cough or change of posture. Some of the diseases they appear in follow.

CHRONIC BRONCHITIS. This condition produces excessive secretion of mucus, resulting in chronic cough productive of sputum. Pathologically, bronchitis is characterized by proliferation and hyperplasia of the mucous glands in the large airways, extending abnormally into small airways, often without evidence of inflammatory changes, although the changes may be associated with bacterial infection. Chronic bronchitis is commonly caused by the inhalation of cigarette smoke, although the disease is found in a few nonsmokers as well, particularly miners and people living in polluted urban environments. The principal complication associated with chronic bronchitis is the development of obstructive airway disease.

ASTHMA. This condition is due to reversible airway obstruction and hyperirritability of the airways. Substances that have no effect when inhaled by nonasthmatic people can cause bronchoconstriction in asthmatics. The severity of asthma is extremely variable, ranging from mild symptoms in children, which may disappear in later life, to severe, continuous, and even fatal obstruction of the airways. Although asthma does not cause emphysema or other chronic diseases, it may itself be a significant cause of disability.

EMPHYSEMA. Emphysema is an abnormal enlargement of the air spaces accompanied by destruction of the alveolar walls, resulting in considerable increase in the volume of the lungs (described more fully in Chapter 1).

Late inspiratory crackles are characteristic of patients with restrictive pulmonary disease (Fig. 5–7). They are usually more numer-

FIGURE 5–7. Phonopneumogram of inspiratory crackles occurring late in inspiration. (From Nath AR, Capel LH: Inspiratory crackles—early and late. *Thorax* 29:223–227, 1974.) (Reprinted by permission of the New England Journal of Medicine.)

ous than early inspiratory crackles, vary with patient position, and are only rarely transmitted to the mouth. They appear to originate in peripheral airways, each crackle representing the abrupt opening of a single airway. Occasionally, late inspiratory crackles are associated with a short end-inspiratory wheeze. These crackles are seen in the following diseases.

INTERSTITIAL FIBROSIS.   This condition, also called interstitial pneumonitis, is associated with interstitial and alveolar infiltrates and fibrosis. Patients complain of cough, of difficulty in breathing, and, rarely, of fever. Pulmonary function studies show restriction and are sensitive indicators of the extent of the illness. Interstitial fibrosis may be caused by cancer chemotherapeutic agents (bleomycin, cyclophosphamide, methotrexate), radiation therapy, the antibiotic nitrofurantoin, high oxygen concentrations inhaled over a long period, and heavy metals such as gold; it is most often idiopathic.

ASBESTOSIS.   Asbestos is widely used in many industries; ship workers, insulators, and people who work with brake linings and asbestos shingles are vulnerable. Inhalation of the tiny asbestos particles leads to pulmonary inflammation and fibrosis. Another disease associated with asbestos exposure, lung cancer, develops particularly among cigarette smokers. People exposed to asbestos also have increased incidence of cancer of the abdominal organs and mesothelioma. Asbestos particles, found in the lungs of nearly all city dwellers, are an extremely potent disease-causing agent; people who have merely worked in shipyards, even if not directly exposed to asbestos, often have asbestos bodies in their lungs and are at high risk to contract lung cancer. In addition, the families of asbestos workers and people living near plants using asbestos have increased risk of lung cancer, which may not occur until 20 or 30 years after exposure.

PNEUMONIA.   An inflammation of the lungs, pneumonia continues to be a major health problem in the United States and, despite antibiotic treatment, an important cause of death. It ranges in severity from a mild illness with a small lung infiltrate visible on chest x-ray to an extensive, progressive, and fatal condition. Pneumonia is most commonly caused by a bacterium, the pneumococcus, but it may be nonbacterial as well—viral, fungal, chemical, or mycoplasmal.

PULMONARY CONGESTION OF HEART FAILURE.   When the left ventricle fails, the lung tissue accumulates excess fluid. Patients complain of progressive shortness of breath, orthopnea, and paroxysmal nocturnal dyspnea.

PULMONARY SARCOIDOSIS.   This is a chronic, often benign disease characterized by noncaseating granulomas in the lung and frequently other parts of the body. It is usually first detected as bilaterally enlarged asymptomatic lymph nodes in the lung hila. The cause is unknown but is believed to be ingestion of a specific substance that provokes an immune reaction. In less than one third of cases, the lung eventually becomes scarred with interstitial fibrosis, leading to restricted pulmonary function.

SCLERODERMA. Scleroderma, more properly called systemic sclerosis or generalized scleroderma, is a disease of connective tissue and is manifested by dermal fibrosis, atrophy of the skin, and fixation of the skin to underlying structures. Systemically, patients develop muscle wasting, joint deformity, diminished esophageal and small bowel function, respiratory insufficiency with pulmonary fibrosis and restriction of lung function, and scleroderma of the kidney followed by renal failure. Scleroderma also frequently affects the heart. The disease affects women three times as frequently as men, with onset usually between the ages of 20 and 55 years. The cause is unknown.

RHEUMATOID LUNG. Rheumatoid arthritis is a systemic disease that causes inflammatory changes in connective tissue throughout the body and commonly damages the smaller joints—proximal interphalangeal, metacarpophalangeal, and metatarsophalangeal. Three times as many women as men are affected and the average age at onset is 35 years. In the lung, the disease causes diffuse interstitial fibrosis, pleural effusions, and nodular lesions. The cause of rheumatoid arthritis is unknown.

Fine and Coarse Crackles

Fine and coarse crackles occur in different lung diseases. Fine crackles are commonly associated with pulmonary fibrosis. Coarse crackles are a characteristic finding in bronchiectasis (discussed in the following section). Time-expanded waveform analysis (Fig. 5–8) demonstrates that the early and late segments of fine and coarse crackles have different characteristics, probably related to the origin of the sound and the resonance of the lung (Munakata et al., 1991).

Figure 5–8 also demonstrates the analysis of fine and coarse crackles by computerized fast Fourier transformation. This mathematical technique transformed a segment of the crackle sound into a spectrum of constituent sound intensities and displays them in relation to sound frequency. Fast Fourier transformation is the most important new procedure for quantifying and analyzing breath sounds. It has been used to study wheezes and transmitted voice sounds, as well as crackles (Anonymous, 1986).

Crackles in Bronchiectasis

Bronchiectasis is a permanent dilatation of the airways that may be very similar to bronchitis. The form of airway enlargement ranges from the generalized cylindric dilatation of chronic bronchitis to sac-

FIGURE 5-8. Example of time-expanded waveform and fast Fourier transform analysis of fine and coarse crackles: (*A*) fine crackle; (*B*) coarse crackle. PF—peak frequency, MF—maximum frequency, IDW—initial deflection width, the duration of the first-half cycle of the crackle waveform; 2CD—the duration of the first two cycles of the crackle waveform; Tb—the duration of the first-quarter cycle of the crackle waveform; Tf—the duration of the first 9/4 cycles of the crackle waveform. (From Munakata M, Ukita H, Doi I, Ohtsuka Y, Masaki Y, Homma Y, Kawakami Y: Spectral and waveform characteristics of fine and coarse crackles. *Thorax* 46:651–657, 1991.)

cular outpouchings from more localized disease. There are many causes of bronchiectasis: airway obstruction by a tumor or foreign body, viral and bacterial pneumonia, tuberculosis, chronic inflammatory or fibrotic pulmonary disease, and heroin-induced pulmonary edema. The crackles of bronchiectasis typically occur in early and midphase inspiration, and airway obstruction is mild (Fig. 5–9); they are coarse and more profuse than most other early inspiratory crackles, are independent of patient position, are usually present in expiration, and become less numerous after coughing. In Table 5–1, the crackles of bronchiectasis are compared with those of other lung diseases.

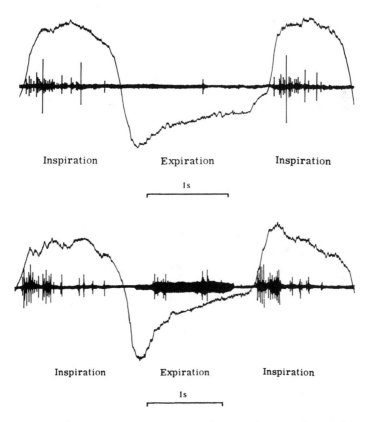

FIGURE 5-9. Phonopneumograms of crackles in bronchiectasis. Patient in upper tracing had chronic bronchitis and bronchiectasis; tracing shows early and midinspiratory crackles. Patient in lower tracing had bronchiectasis and lung fibrosis; pan-inspiratory and expiratory crackles are seen. Lung crackles here are more profuse in early and midinspiration. (From Nath AR, Capel LH: Lung crackles in bronchiectasis. *Thorax* 35:694–699, 1980.)

TABLE 5-1.   Crackles in various lung diseases*

Condition	Associated Crackles
Healthy	Fine crackles at anterior bases, only during inspiration from low lung volume
Idiopathic interstitial fibrosis	Prominent fine crackles
Asbestosis	Prominent fine crackles, may be first indication of disease
Bronchiectasis	Coarse crackles, often heard at the mouth
Chronic bronchitis	Coarse crackles, often heard at the mouth
Congestive heart failure	Fine crackles
Sarcoidosis	Sparse fine crackles
Miliary tuberculosis	Sparse fine crackles
Other granulomatous lung diseases	Sparse fine crackles

(From Kraman SS: Lung sounds for the clinician. *Arch Int Med* 146:1411–1412, 1986. Copyright 1986, American Medical Association.)

*For a description of identifiable characteristics of fine and coarse crackles, see text.

Crackles are not necessarily an abnormal finding. For example, Thacker and Kraman were able to record crackles anteriorly in 26 of 52 normal subjects (mostly male) when they inhaled deeply from residual volume. These crackles were commonly profuse and loud. Wave form analysis showed them to be like the crackles of interstitial lung disease (Thacker and Kraman, 1982). Workum has obtained similar results in normal women (Workum et al., 1982). Both groups found these crackles to be very rarely, if ever, heard during breathing from resting lung volume.

The incidence of crackles is important in the diagnosis of pulmonary disease. For example, Epler has reported that bilateral high-pitched crackles are heard in 60 percent of patients with interstitial pneumonias and asbestosis but in only 20 percent of those with sarcoidosis and other granulomatoses (Epler et al., 1978) (Figs. 5–10 and 5–11). In asbestosis, high-pitched crackles correlated with pathologic severity, with honeycombing changes in the lung on x-ray, and with physiologic abnormalities. Furthermore, the presence of bilateral basal crackles is closely related to the duration of asbestos exposure; these crackles often occur before asbestosis is detected on chest x-ray (Shirai et al., 1981) (Fig. 5–12). Therefore, although crackles are not always abnormal, they should be listened for in a patient with a history suggestive of disease.

Crackles should also be searched for in patients who have just suffered a myocardial infarction. Crackles that appear over the upper two thirds of the posterior lung fields, while the patient is still in the coro-

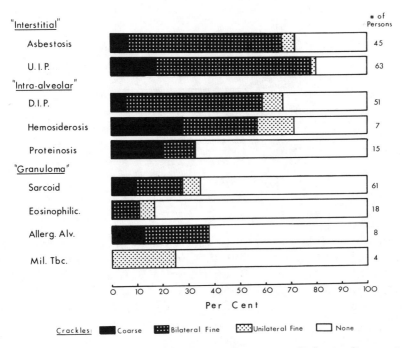

FIGURE 5–10. Types of crackles according to pathologic diagnosis in 272 patients with chronic infiltrative pulmonary disease diagnosed by biopsy. U.I.P., unusual interstitial pneumonia; D.I.P., desquamative interstitial pneumonia; Allerg. Alv., allergic alveolitis; Mil. Tbc., miliary tuberculosis. (From Epler GR, Carrington CB, Gaensler EA: Crackles (rales) in the interstitial pulmonary diseases. *Chest* 73:333–339, 1978.)

nary care unit, are an extremely bad sign. A patient with such crackles is 3.3 times more likely to die in the 2-year period following the infarct than is the same patient without these crackles. Crackles heard only at the lung bases—that is, the lower third of the posterior lung fields—do not have the same dire significance.

The exact cardiac abnormality that causes the crackles over the upper two thirds of the posterior lung fields is as yet uncertain. Surprisingly, they are unrelated to radionuclide ejection fraction, a technique used to assess the function of the left ventricle (The Multicenter Postinfarction Research Group, 1983).

Wheezes

A wheeze (rhonchus) is a musical pulmonary sound. The musical character, obvious to any listener, is determined by the spectrum of fre-

FIGURE 5-11.   Incidence and types of crackles according to clinical diagnoses in 657 patients. Note that crackles were most common in asbestosis.   (From Epler GR, Carrington CB, Gaensler EA: Crackles (rales) in the interstitial pulmonary diseases. *Chest* 73:333–339, 1978.)

FIGURE 5-12.   Bilateral basal crackles and radiographic abnormalities in asbestos workers—relationship between prevalence and duration of exposure. Note that crackles occurred before radiographic abnormalities.   (From Shirai F, Kudoh S, Shibuya A, et al.: Crackles in asbestos workers: Auscultation and lung sound analysis. *Br J Dis Chest* 75:386–396, 1981.)

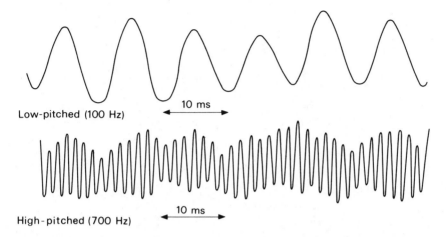

Low-pitched (100 Hz)

10 ms

High-pitched (700 Hz)

10 ms

FIGURE 5-13. Wave forms of a wheeze. The musical character of the wheezing sound can be recognized by the regular pattern formed by a sequence of identical wave forms. (From Forgacs P: *Lung Sounds.* London, Baillière Tindall, 1978.)

quencies that make up the sound. The lowest or fundamental frequency sets the pitch of the note.

The musical character of the wheezing sound can be recognized on a phonopneumogram by the regular pattern formed by a sequence of identical wave forms (Fig. 5-13). Wheezes are classified as high- or low-pitched, inspiratory or expiratory, short or long, and single or multiple. A monophonic wheeze consists of a single note or of several notes starting and ending at different times. A polyphonic wheeze is made up of several dissonant notes starting and ending simultaneously, like a chord.

The most widely accepted mechanism of wheezing, described by Dr. Paul Forgacs, is analogous to a vibrating reed. The reed produces a sound that is identical to that of a bronchus narrowed to the point of closure, whose opposite walls oscillate between the closed and barely open positions. When the caliber of a bronchus is reduced to the point of closure and a musical note of constant pitch is generated, this pitch is unaffected by the density of the ambient gas. The detached mouthpiece of an oboe or the reed of a child's toy trumpet behaves in the same way (Fig. 5-14).

The vibrating reed mechanism makes it incorrect to attribute high-pitched wheezing to short peripheral airways and low-pitched wheezing to long central bronchi. It is true that the oscillations of a large mass, such as a tumor occluding a main bronchus, usually produce a low-pitched note. Nevertheless, high-pitched wheezing may be generated centrally or peripherally and may rise or fall during a single respiratory cycle in parallel with the tightness of the compression.

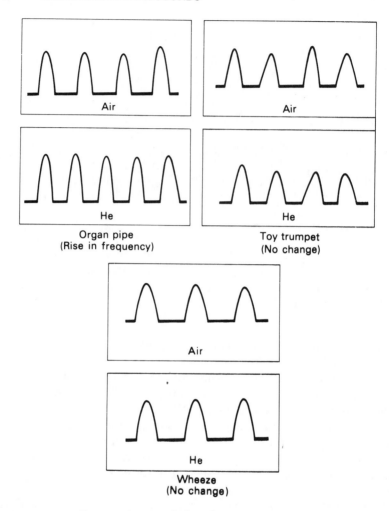

FIGURE 5–14. Comparison of the frequency of wind instruments blown with air or helium (He) and a wheeze when air or oxygen and helium are inhaled. Note that the frequency of the organ pipe rises when blown with helium, but that of a toy trumpet and a wheeze do not change. This indicates that a wheeze is produced by a vibrating reed-type mechanism that, like the vibrating reed in the toy trumpet, is unaffected by the density of the ambient gas. (From Forgacs P: *Lung Sounds*. London, Baillière Tindall, 1978.)

For many years, investigators believed that the musical sound of wheezing was generated in a manner similar to sound production within an organ pipe. The gas within a narrowed bronchus was supposed to be set into oscillation in much the same way as a stream of air blown across a flue pipe, producing a musical note whose pitch was determined by the dimensions of the pipe. Thus, a simple reduction in the pipe caliber or a spur facing the stream of gas in the airway was assumed sufficient to generate musical sounds; the pitch of the note would depend on the length of the adjoining airway. High-pitched wheezing was therefore often attributed to peripheral bronchial spasm.

Although this theory of wheezing may be attractive, it is contradicted by several facts: (1) The longest axial pathway in the bronchial tree is less than 1 foot, whereas the frequency of some low-pitched wheezes is in the range produced by pipes 4 to 8 feet long. (2) Unlike the sound of an organ pipe, the pitch of a wheeze emanating from a stenosed bronchus is not fixed; indeed, it may differ by as much as an octave between inspiration and expiration. In experiments with excised bronchi, no musical sound results from a simple reduction in caliber until the opposite walls of the compressed bronchus are brought into contact. The frequency of the note can then be varied over several octaves by tightening the compression or increasing the blowing pressure. (3) The definitive argument against the organ pipe model is that the pitch of the tone rises when the pipe is blown with helium, a less dense gas than air. However, the pitch of a wheeze stays constant when the inspired air is replaced by a mixture of helium and oxygen (Forgacs, 1978b).

Monophonic Wheezes

A characteristic example of a monophonic wheeze is the single musical tone made by a bronchus that is almost completely occluded by tumor. If the narrowing is rigid, the wheeze can be heard throughout the respiratory cycle; if the narrowing is flexible, the wheeze may not be audible during either inspiration or expiration, especially if the patient is turned from one side to the other. Single or multiple monophonic wheezes are a characteristic clinical sign of asthma. The number of wheezes is never large; the illusion that many wheezes are heard under the stethoscope results from the wide transmission of a few loud wheezes with varying relative intensity to different points on the chest wall.

In asbestosis and interstitial fibrosis, an unusual type of monophonic wheezing is occasionally heard over the lower regions of the lung. It is restricted to inspiration and is often associated with late inspiratory crackling. Some of these patients have a single short wheeze at the end of inspiration; others have several short wheezes of different pitch following one another throughout inspiration.

As was mentioned, late inspiratory crackles and an end-inspiratory wheeze are often associated. That both are heard over deflated regions of the lung suggests that their mode of production is similar. Apparently, end-inspiratory wheezes are produced by airways, the walls of which oscillate in apposition for a few milliseconds before opening fully. Because these airways open at a predetermined transpulmonary pressure, the same sequence of musical notes will occur in several consecutive respiratory cycles (Forgacs, 1978b).

Polyphonic Wheezes

Polyphonic wheezing is a frequent sign of most types of chronic obstructive pulmonary disease. It is confined largely to expiration and, as was mentioned, is composed of several dissonant notes starting and ending at the same time.

A polyphonic wheeze is produced by compression of the central bronchi. Although it is a reliable sign of widespread obstruction to air flow, polyphonic wheezing can also be generated in normal subjects, in whom it is called a forced expiratory wheeze (Kraman, 1983). There are two ways to differentiate a forced expiratory wheeze from a pathologic polyphonic wheeze.

1. A forced expiratory wheeze can be produced in normal subjects only during a violent expiratory effort. In contrast, patients with severe air flow obstruction will wheeze even during a gentle expiration.

2. In a healthy subject, during a forced expiration, the progressively louder breath sounds will retain their character as *white noise* until a strong expiratory effort, delivered with maximum force, suddenly evokes the full complement of musical sounds contained in the forced expiratory wheeze. (As was pointed out in Chapter 4, white noise is made up of sound waves of many different frequencies and is analogous to white light, which is composed of light waves of many different frequencies.) In contrast, subjects with diseased lungs will produce a sequence of musical sounds, starting with a monophonic wheeze at a mildly forced expiration and progressing to bitonal and multiple wheezes with increased effort; the full polyphonic wheeze will eventually follow (Forgacs, 1978b).

Polyphonic wheezing is heard in all forms of obstructive lung disease, asthma and emphysema being examples. An abnormal polyphonic wheeze is the direct result of pathologic changes that have taken place within the bronchi. In contrast, the forced expiratory wheeze does not result from pathologic changes—simply from a high rate of air flow.

Stridor and Hoarseness

Stridor is a particularly loud musical sound of constant pitch, most prominent during inspiration, and heard very well at a distance from the patient. Although nothing except its intensity distinguishes stridor from a monophonic wheeze, which cannot be heard at a distance from the patient, the term is widely used when laryngeal or tracheal obstruction is known or suspected to be the source of the sound (Forgacs, 1978b).

The mechanism of stridor, like that of wheezing, is analogous to a vibrating reed. The reed will produce a sound that is identical to a larynx or trachea narrowed to the point of closure, the opposite walls of which oscillate between the closed and barely open positions; they all produce a musical note of constant pitch. However, stridor is generated in central airways, whereas wheezing comes from more peripheral airways.

Though stridor is typically inspiratory, it becomes inspiratory and expiratory as the airway becomes increasingly obstructed, as by laryngeal tumors, tracheal stenosis, or an aspirated foreign body. When particularly severe, stridor is associated with gasping respiration and use of the accessory muscles of respiration.

Hoarseness is a roughened, coarse quality of the voice, occurring whenever a normal, smooth vocal cord is not brought into contact with its fellow. Hoarseness indicates either that there are irregularities on the surface of one or both cords or that there is a disorder of nerves and muscles responsible for vocal cord movement. Hoarseness is dealt with in this section because, although not a wheeze, it can be produced by the same pathologic changes in the larynx that cause stridor.

Hoarseness and stridor have very different significance in children and adults. The diseases causing these conditions are discussed in the following section.

Stridor in Children

In a child, obstruction of the airway and trachea is usually much more rapid and life-threatening than in an adult. Severe obstruction is accompanied by cyanosis and pallor of the skin, dilatation of the nostrils, downward plunging of the trachea, and use of the accessory muscles of respiration. Voice changes, swallowing difficulties, respiratory infections, and failure to thrive are seen in less severe obstruction (Ludman, 1981). There are several causes of airway obstruction in a child.

Laryngomalacia (congenital stridor) is manifested in the first few months of life. Characteristically, the infant appears to be normal except for the stridor, which is particularly audible when the infant is supine or excited. Laryngomalacia means softening of the larynx; this, in fact, is what one sees through the laryngoscope. The epiglottis, arytenoid cartilage, and aryepiglottic folds are "floppy" and drawn into the larynx during inspiration. The condition commonly becomes more severe during the first year of life but then gradually improves, with complete recovery.

Viral croup is the most common cause of upper airway obstruction in infants. Most cases occur between October and April in children

FIGURE 5-15. A hospital croup tent that is used to treat children with viral croup. (From Valman HB: Stridor. *Brit Med J* 283:294–295, 1981.)

3 months to 3 years of age, and boys outnumber girls 2 to 1. The signs and symptoms usually begin suddenly at night, after several days of upper respiratory infection. The child has stridor and a characteristic barking, croupy cough; anxiety worsens the problem. Tracheostomy or intubation is performed in severe cases; the mortality rate may be as high as 2.7 percent. Humidity administered by vaporizer, racemic epinephrine by aerosol, steam inhalation at home, and "croup tent" in the hospital (Fig. 5–15) are the most common forms of treatment (Anonymous, 1987; Roberts, 1979).

Acute epiglottitis (Fig. 5–16) is a severe, often fatal infection caused by *Hemophilus influenzae* type B bacteria. The illness develops very rapidly. After a few hours of sore throat and fever, the child's jaw protrudes; he drools, refuses to swallow, and appears anxious. The stridor and other signs result from swelling of the epiglottis and upper portion of the larynx. Mortality can be reduced from 24 percent to 2 percent by provision of an airway through nasotracheal intubation or tracheostomy. At present, chloramphenicol is the antibiotic of choice. Epiglottitis is ordinarily a brief illness; most patients need the airway for a day or two at most.

Diphtheria, caused by *Corynebacterium diphtheriae*, is quite rare today. Nevertheless, it should be suspected if a dirty gray, tough, fibrinous pseudomembrane is present in the throat in the region of the tonsils. As the disease progresses, swelling of the pharynx and larynx obstructs breathing. When untreated, death may result from complete, sudden airway obstruction or from heart failure, the result of a toxin produced by the bacteria. Diphtheria antitoxin and antibiotics—procaine penicillin, ampicillin, erythromycin, clindamycin, or rifampin—are an effective form of therapy (Berkow, 1977). With immunization, the diphtheria epidemics of past centuries have all but disappeared.

RADIOGRAPHIC APPEARANCES

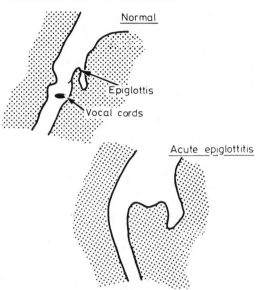

FIGURE 5–16. Appearance of the larynx in normal children and in those with acute epiglottitis. Note the swelling of the epiglottis in the latter condition. (From Valman HB: Stridor. *Brit Med J* 283:294–295, 1981.)

Medical historians speculate that one such epidemic caused the death of George Washington in 1799.

Laryngeal paralysis at birth is believed to result from the stretching of the vagus nerve during a difficult delivery. The condition is associated with feeding difficulties. The child may prefer to lie with the head turned to one side, and there may be unilateral facial weakness. Spontaneous recovery occurs during the first year of life.

Congenital narrowing of the larynx or trachea may be caused by webs between the cords or by narrowing of the space beneath (Fig. 5–17). Surgical correction is often necessary.

Inhalation of a foreign body causes 3000 Americans to choke to death annually. Foreign body obstruction of the adult airway frequently occurs while the victim is eating. In a child, choking may occur during play, when a small toy or object being mouthed slips back into the airway. There are four signs of choking: (1) inability to speak or breathe, (2) pallor followed by increasing cyanosis, (3) loss of consciousness and collapse, and (4) the so-called Heimlich sign, in which the victim brings his hand to his throat with the thumb and index finger spread wide to form a "V." The foreign body may be dislodged by the Heimlich maneuver (Fig. 5–18).

Stridor and Hoarseness in Adults

In an adult, abnormalities of the larynx cause hoarseness more often than they cause stridor. Acute hoarseness, a change in the voice

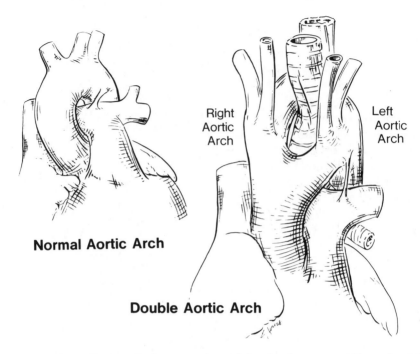

Normal Aortic Arch

Right Aortic Arch

Left Aortic Arch

Double Aortic Arch

FIGURE 5-17.   Congenital narrowing of the trachea caused by a double aortic arch.

of less than 3 weeks' duration, may be caused by infectious laryngitis; trauma from shouting, coughing, or vomiting; inhalation of smoke or noxious fumes; or allergic swelling (angioedema). Chronic hoarseness—hoarseness of more than 3 weeks' duration—may be due to the following conditions.

Chronic laryngitis, a continuing irritation of the laryngeal mucosa, is often a result of straining the voice during an acute attack of laryngitis, with submucosal hemorrhage and vocal cord edema. Tuberculosis and syphilis are uncommon causes. Vocal cord nodules (singer's nodules) develop after chronic voice abuse such as screaming or shouting. They are tiny fibrous nodules of both vocal cords and may be removed surgically.

Vocal cord paralysis is frequently caused by damage to the recurrent laryngeal nerve. The damage is often inflicted by a cancer in the hilum of the lung. Sometimes the nerve is injured during thyroidectomy or is affected by neuritis. In many cases, no cause is found.

Neoplasms of the larynx may arise from the vocal cords (glottic), or from above or below them (supraglottic, subglottic) (Fig. 5-19). Malignant tumors are almost invariably squamous cell carcinomas and are more common in men than in women. The patient gives a history of years of smoking cigarettes. The chance of survival is greatest in vocal cord carcinomas, which cause hoarseness very early and spread to the lymph nodes in the neck only after a long period of growth. Subglottic carcinomas have the worst prognosis. Carcinoma of the pyriform fossa invades the muscles of the larynx and causes hoarseness late in the disease.

Any patient with more than 3 weeks of hoarseness should be examined by indirect laryngoscopy. Most laryngeal tumors can be seen with a mirror. A biopsy is then obtained by direct laryngoscopy under general anesthesia. Other diagnostic methods employed include x-ray laryngography with contrast medium and laryngeal tomography.

Chronic laryngitis is treated by resting of the voice and elimination of irritants, by humidification of the home, and by steam inhalation. Cancer of the larynx is treated by surgery, external irradiation, and chemotherapy; the modality or combination of modalities employed depends on the extent of the disease.

In an adult, airway obstruction may be caused by large tumors, bilateral paralysis of laryngeal nerves, or inhalation of foreign bodies, particularly lumps of food. The physician can quickly relieve laryngeal obstruction by making an incision over the cricothyroid membrane and inserting a tube. Because the cricothyroid membrane is just below the skin surface, this procedure, called laryngotomy (Fig. 5–20), is much more simply and safely performed than is a tracheostomy. The treatment of choice for inhaled food is the Heimlich maneuver (Fig 5–18).

Sometimes, an adult may experience airway obstruction that lacks an identifiable organic cause. Such patients have dramatic episodes of stridor, which may have been mistaken for asthma and ordinary wheezing. The stridor results from complete adduction of the true vocal cords, reducing the glottic opening to a small posterior diamond-shaped chink. People with this condition show a variety of psychiatric disorders, ranging from mild stress-related worsening of symptoms to obsessive-compulsive neurosis; they have difficulty in directly expressing anger, sadness, or fear and have various degrees of secondary gain from their respiratory symptoms. Treatment consists of teaching the patients to concentrate on active expiration by using their ventral abdominal muscles and to relax the oropharyngeal muscles. In combination with short-term psychotherapy, these measures immediately reduce both the number and severity of attacks in all patients (Christopher, 1983).

Pleural Friction Rub

The smooth, moist layers of the normal pleura move easily and silently over one another. However, when the surface is coarsened by fibrin

Infant is either held in rescuer's lap or placed face up on a firm surface with the rescuer at his feet. Rescuer places index and middle fingers of both hands on child's abdomen, slightly above navel and well below the rib cage, and presses into abdomen with a *quick upward thrust*. Several thrusts may be necessary to expel the object

FIGURE 5–18.   The Heimlich maneuver. (*A*) An infant victim.

deposits or thickened by inflammatory or neoplastic cells, the sliding motion is impeded by frictional resistance. The sound produced resembles that of a stringed instrument; if a large area of the chest wall is involved, the sound is musical.

More commonly, however, the irregular sliding movement of the lung generates a series of nonmusical sounds, usually longer and of lower pitch than lung crackles; a characteristic pleural friction rub has been compared to the creaking sound of old leather (Fig. 5–21).

A distinctive feature of a pleural friction rub is that the sound, audible during inspiration, frequently recurs in reverse sequence during expiration; Forgacs refers to this as the "mirror image effect." Sometimes, the crackling sound made by a very high-pitched rub is indistinguishable from a crackle emanating from within the lung. In

B

1. Rescuer stands behind victim and wraps his arms around victim's waist

2. Rescuer makes a fist with one hand and places the thumb side of the fist against the victim's abdomen, slightly above the navel and below the rib cage

3. Rescuer grasps fist with other hand and presses into victim's abdomen with a *quick upward thrust*

4. Thrust is repeated several times if necessary

C

Victim on back with face up. Facing victim, rescuer kneels astride victim's hips. Rescuer then places his hands one on top of the other with the heel of the bottom hand on victim's abdomen, slightly above the navel and below the rib cage. He presses into abdomen with a *quick upward thrust*. Thrust repeated several times if necessary

FIGURE 5–18. *Continued.* (*B*) Victim standing. (*C*) Victim supine. (© Copyright 1979, CIBA Pharmaceutical Company, Division of CIBA-GEIGY Corporation. Reprinted with permission from CLINICAL SYMPOSIA, illustrated by Frank H. Netter, M.D. All rights reserved.)

115

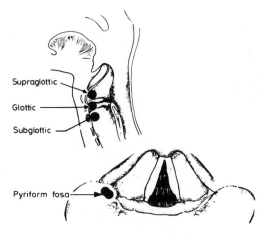

FIGURE 5-19. The larynx seen in cross section from the side and from above. Tumors may arise from the pyriform fossa or from the subglottic, glottic, or supraglottic regions. (From Ludman H: Hoarseness and stridor. *Brit Med J* 282:715–717, 1981.)

this case, differentiation is made on the basis of circumstantial evidence (Forgacs, 1978b); also, a rub is not affected by coughing.

Mediastinal Crunch (Hamman's Sign)

The mediastinal crunch is a coarse, crackling sound or vibration that is synchronous with systole and is frequently heard over the precordium in the presence of mediastinal emphysema. The air within the mediastinum producing the crunch may be present in trauma patients or patients who have undergone cardiopulmonary resuscitation. The distinctive crunching or popping sound is believed to result from air separating the visceral and parietal pericardium during contraction of the heart; sometimes, the crunching may also be due to left pneumothorax and gas in close contact with the heart or to elevation of the left hemidiaphragm caused by air in the fundus of the stomach.

FIGURE 5-20. Diagram of the neck, showing where incisions for tracheostomy and laryngotomy are made to relieve airway obstruction. (From Ludman H: Hoarseness and stridor. *Brit Med J* 282:715–717, 1981.)

FIGURE 5-21.   Pleural friction rub. Note the bursts of sound occurring in rapid succession.   (From McKusick VA: *Cardiovascular Sound in Health and Disease.* Baltimore, Williams & Wilkins, 1958.)

Bronchial Leak Squeak

The bronchial leak squeak is a physical diagnostic sign in patients with bronchopleurocutaneous fistula. This sound is heard as a high pitched squeak over the affected chest area during sustained Valsalva maneuver, the pitch being higher in smaller fistulas than in larger fistulas. Decreases in intensity and increases in pitch occur in patients whose bronchial fistulas close slowly. When the leak squeak sign is absent in patients with spontaneous pneumothorax, one may assume that alveoli, rather than central airways, are leaking (Krumpe et al., 1981).

Inspiratory Squawk

A distinctive inspiratory musical sound, called a squawk, is found in some patients with diffuse pulmonary fibrosis (Earis et al., 1982). Allergic inflammation of the alveoli, also called hypersensitivity pneumonitis, appears to predispose to squawks.

Hypersensitivity pneumonitis results from the inhalation of organic antigens in susceptible individuals. The condition was initially described as "farmer's lung" and occurred after the inhalation of moldy hay contaminated by fungal organisms. Subsequently, many hobbies, occupations, and living conditions have been associated with this entity. Those affected include bird fanciers, detergent workers, mushroom pickers, cheese workers, and others. Maple bark, wood pulp, cork dust, coffee beans, redwood sawdust, and other substances have been demonstrated to cause the condition; some may be contaminated by fungi, but often no fungus is involved.

Generally, the squawks of allergic alveolitis are of shorter duration, occur later in inspiration, and tend to be of higher pitch than those

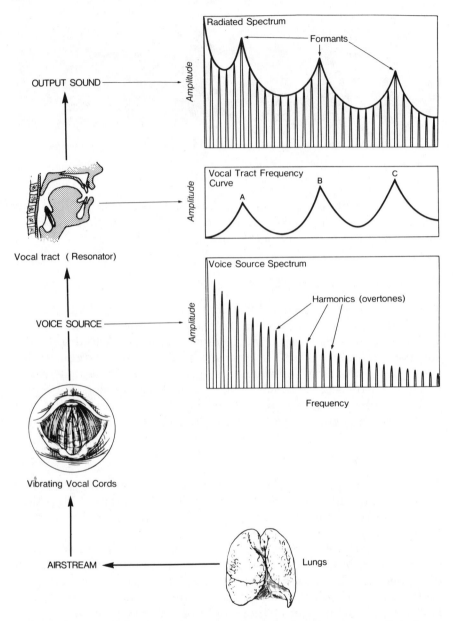

FIGURE 5–22. Voice sounds are produced when a stream of air from the lungs is periodically interrupted by the vibrating vocal cords. The resulting sound, the voice source, has a spectrum composed of a large number of harmonics, also called overtones. The vocal tract—the larynx, pharynx, nose, and mouth—is a resonator, that is, it has characteristic frequencies or formants (A, B, C) that it transmits best. As the voice source moves through the vocal tract, each harmonic is attenu-

heard in pulmonary fibrosis of nonallergic origin. The squawk is almost invariably accompanied by inspiratory crackles. Like the crackles, the squawk seems to result from the opening of airways.

ABNORMALLY TRANSMITTED SOUNDS

Egophony

Egophony (Greek: the voice of a goat) refers to the nasal or bleating quality of speech transmitted through consolidated lung tissue (as, for example, in pneumonia) or occasionally over a pleural effusion, when the effusion causes collapse and atelectasis of underlying lung.

When voice sounds are transmitted to the chest wall through consolidated lung tissue, the normal sound filtering of the lung is diminished and, as a result, the higher frequencies are enhanced. Such a transmutation of the sound produces the phenomenon known as "E to A egophony" (McKusick et al., 1955).

The raw material for speech, called the voice source, is the sound generated by the airstream chopped by the vocal cords. It is a complex tone composed of a fundamental frequency (determined by the vibratory frequency of the vocal cords) and a large number of higher pitched harmonics, also called overtones.

The vocal tract—the larynx, pharynx, nose, and mouth—is a resonator; in other words, it has certain frequencies that it transmits best. The four or five most important of these frequencies are called *formants*. The closer a tone generated by the vocal cords is to the formant frequency, the louder it will be transmitted (Fig. 5–22).

Figure 5–23 shows sound spectrograms of the letters E and A when spoken into a microphone. As can be seen, E lacks the higher frequencies or formants associated with A.

In Figure 5–24, the spectrogram on the left shows the normal letter E recorded through the chest wall. Notice the very prominent low-

ated in proportion to its distance from the formant nearest it in frequency. The formant frequencies thus appear as peaks in the spectrum of sound radiated from the lips. The peaks establish particular vowel sounds. The higher peaks are not normally transmitted to the chest wall, thus rendering spoken words unintelligible through the stethoscope under ordinary conditions. However, the higher frequencies are transmitted through consolidated lung tissue in conditions such as pneumonia, rendering speech intelligible over the chest wall through a stethoscope. (Adapted from Sundberg J: The acoustics of the singing voice. *Scientific American* 236(3):82–91, March 1977.)

FIGURE 5-23. The spectrogram of the sounds "E" and "A" when spoken directly into the microphone. Note that "A" is composed of many more high-frequency components or formants than "E." (From McKusick VA, Jenkins JT, Webb GN: The acoustic basis of the chest examination. Studies by means of sound spectrography. *Am Rev Tuber* 72:12–34, 1955.)

est formant at about 180 Hz. The spectrogram on the right shows the E to A change when heard through the consolidated lung of a patient with pneumonia. Notice that the upper frequencies have been enhanced, making the spoken E sound like A.

This phenomenon appears to have been discovered simultaneously in 1922, by Shibley in China (Shibley, 1922) and Froschels in Vienna (Froschels and Stockert, 1922). Shibley reported that five vowel sounds—A, E, I, O, U—all became "A" or "Ah," both over a localized

FIGURE 5-24.   "E" to "A" egophony. Note the very prominent lowest formant of "E" (arrow) at about 180 Hz in the spectrogram on the left. The spectrogram on the right shows the "E" to "A" change when heard through the consolidated lung of a patient with pneumonia. Note that the higher frequencies have been enhanced, making the spoken "E" sound like "A." (From McKusick VA, Jenkins JT, Webb GN: The acoustic basis of the chest examination. Studies by means of sound spectrography. *Am Rev Tuberc* 72:12–34, 1955.)

area of fluid or consolidation and over a large goiter. He came upon the sign accidentally, while having his Chinese patients say "i, er, san" (one, two, three). The word for "one" was pronounced "E" in his province; thus, the origin of the E to A sign. Froschels reported that one vowel sound might be changed into another with no particular predictability.

To elicit egophony, the examiner should place the bell of the stethoscope over each point on the chest wall corresponding to a bronchopulmonary segment (see Chapter 4). The patient should be asked to say the letter "E" over and over. If an "A"-like sound is perceived, then the patient has egophony.

Whispered Pectoriloquy

During whispering, the vocal cords do not oscillate; voice sounds are generated by the turbulent flow of air through the trachea, glottis, and pharynx. This white noise is missing the prominent low-frequency oscillations (below 200 Hz) of normal voice sounds and is therefore much softer than normal speech.

Whispered sounds, which lack the low frequencies best transmitted by air-containing lung, are inaudible over the normal chest. However, through airless consolidated lung tissue, the high-pitched sounds (above 200 Hz) are transmitted, and the whispering becomes audible (Fig. 5–25). This sign is called whispered pectoriloquy.

To elicit whispered pectoriloquy, the stethoscope should be

FIGURE 5-25.   Whispered pectoriloquy. Note that in pneumonia, the spectrogram indicates that the higher frequencies in the words *one, two, three* have been transmitted, while in the normal subject they have not. The transmission of these higher frequencies makes the words intelligible through a stethoscope over the chest wall. (From McKusick VA, Jenkins JT, Webb GN: The acoustic basis of the chest examination. Studies by means of sound spectrography. *Am Rev Tuberc* 72:12–34, 1955.)

placed over each bronchopulmonary segment. The patient should be asked to whisper "one, two, three." If the words are clearly audible over one segment, then the segment is designated as showing whispered pectoriloquy. The examiner should listen for whispered pectoriloquy with great care, as it is in general more difficult to identify than other abnormal sounds, such as wheezing (Spitter et al., 1988).

Bronchophony and Bronchial Breathing

As the result of the selective transmission of sound through normal lung, the higher frequencies and most of the vowel formants are lost; speech heard through the stethoscope becomes a meaningless, low pitched mumble. However, when lung between the stethoscope and the trachea is airless, the higher frequencies and vowel formants are transmitted. As a result, speech becomes clear, a sign called *bronchophony*. Likewise, high-pitched breath sounds are transmitted through consolidated lung tissue to the chest wall in *bronchial breathing* (Fig. 5–26).

Bronchophony and bronchial breathing are both signs of the unfiltered transmission of sounds through consolidated lung tissue; they are produced by the same mechanism as whispered pectoriloquy. For bronchial breathing to occur, consolidated lung tissue must extend at least 3 to 5 cm from the chest wall, except near the vertebral column, where it must be 1 to 2 cm from the surface (Martini and Müller, 1923; McKusick et al., 1955).

To elicit bronchophony, the examiner should place the stethoscope over each bronchopulmonary segment. The patient should be asked to say "ninety-nine." If these words are clearly audible and not a meaningless jumble, then bronchophony is said to be present.

Important note: All of the foregoing diagnostic signs—egophony, whispered pectoriloquy, bronchophony, and bronchial breathing—are the result of one thing: sound transmission through airless lung with resulting loss of normal filtering. They all have the same significance. Moreover, having the patient say "one, two, three" or "ninety-nine" is only a convention; in fact, bronchophony and whispered pectoriloquy could be elicited just as well if the patient said almost anything.

Poor Breath Sounds with Good Voice Sounds

In patients with bronchial stenosis, the breath sounds over the involved lung are faint or absent, whereas the voice sounds are normal (Fig. 5–26). This sign is applicable only to stenosis of the main, intermediate, or lobar bronchi (Jones, 1988).

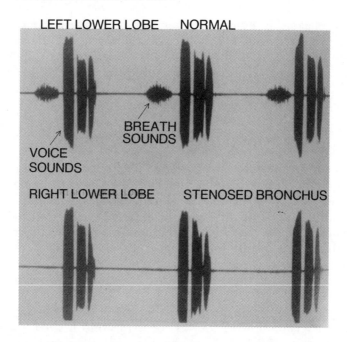

FIGURE 5-26. Simultaneous recordings of breath sounds and voice sounds at corresponding sites over the left lower lobe (normal bronchus) and right lower lobe (stenosed bronchus). Patient inspired deeply, spoke words "three, four, eight," and then exhaled. Three consecutive breaths are shown. Note that breath sounds are absent over the right lower lobe, which was stenosed. Note also that voice sounds were well transmitted on both sides. (From Jones FL: Poor breath sounds with good voice sounds. A sign of bronchial stenosis. *Chest* 93:312–313, 1988.)

Noisy Breathing at the Mouth

One of the most useful signs of chronic obstructive pulmonary disease is noisy breathing (Forgacs, 1978a). The breathing of most patients with chronic bronchitis or asthma is noisy, whereas the breath sounds of a healthy subject cannot be heard at a distance of a few centimeters from the mouth, unless he is panting, gasping, or sighing. The breathing of many patients with chronic obstructive pulmonary disease is accompanied by a noise that can be heard across the room. This noise is not to be confused with the adventitious sounds already discussed.

Forgacs has measured the noise during inspiration and confirmed the clinical observation that the loudness of the inspiratory breath sounds heard close to the patient's mouth reflects the severity of obstruction to the flow of air. The source of the noise appears to be turbulence in the gas flowing through the airways.

RELATIONSHIP OF BREATH SOUND INTENSITY TO VENTILATORY FUNCTION

Since the nineteenth century, medical writings have referred to a reduction in the loudness of breath sounds over the chest as evidence for the presence of emphysema. This observation has been tested on a quantitative basis by Pardee (Pardee et al., 1976) and Bohadana (Bohadana et al., 1978). Diminished breath sounds correlated quite well with diminished percentage of predicted forced expiratory volume in one second (FEV_1) as well as with other measurements of obstruction and vital capacity. In other words, patients with emphysema and very faint breath sounds will probably have very poor pulmonary function. Indeed, patients with severe emphysema often have practically no detectable lung sounds at all. A useful, quantitative way to test for the loudness of breath sounds is by obtaining a breath sound score. To obtain this score, auscultation is performed at the following six locations: bilaterally over the upper anterior portion of the chest, in the midaxillae, and at the posterior bases. Breath sound intensity is estimated in inspiration during a response to the request that the subject take a deep breath with his mouth open. The loudness of the sounds is scaled in five stages: 0—silent, 1—barely audible, 2—faint but definitely heard breath sounds, 3—expected for normal, and 4—louder than usual normal. The numerical grades for the six areas sampled are added to give a total breath sound score. The score can then be compared to the following table to obtain a crude approximation of FEV_1/FVC (see Chapter 1 for the significance of this measurement):

Total Breath Sound Score	FEV_1/FVC (%)
10	27
12	38
14	49
16	60
18	71
20	82

Example: A 55-year-old white man, a heavy smoker, was examined. The examiner obtained the following scores:

Location	Breath Sound Score
Right upper anterior chest	3
Left upper anterior chest	2
Right midaxilla	2
Left midaxilla	3
Right posterior base	3
Left posterior base	1
Total breath sound score	14

From the table on page 125, the patient in the example with a total breath sound score of 14 has an FEV_1/FVC of 49 percent.

SLEEP APNEA SYNDROME

During sleep, people with sleep apnea periodically stop breathing. Many normal people stop breathing 10 times a night or less for a period of less than 20 seconds. However, a person with sleep apnea may stop breathing once or twice every minute; this adds up to almost 1000 apneas over 8 hours, each of which may last from 10 to more than 60 seconds.

Patients with sleep apnea complain most commonly of excessive daytime sleepiness, but they also may note insomnia. A spouse or bedmate will complain of their loud, excessive snoring. Sleep apnea may be classified as two types, obstructive and nonobstructive.

Obstructive sleep apnea is due to a periodic obstruction within the upper airway, usually in an obese male with a thick neck. The definitive treatment for this condition is a tracheostomy, which creates a bypass below the upper airway obstruction. For obstructive sleep apneas that are not severe enough to warrant a tracheostomy, one experimental form of treatment is the placement of a mask that fits over the face and is worn at night to provide a positive pressure on the airway and thus keep it open.

Nonobstructive sleep apnea results from an abnormality of the respiratory center in the pons, a section of the brain near the medulla. The abnormality may be due to vascular disease, meningitis, encephalitis, or tumor or may be of unknown cause. Breathing is normal, without apnea, in the awake patient, because the inadequacy of the respiratory center is compensated for by other impulses moving through the cortical tracts of the brain. However, during sleep, when cortical impulses cease, the respiratory center is insufficient to maintain regular respiration. Tracheostomy is of no value in nonobstructive sleep apnea.

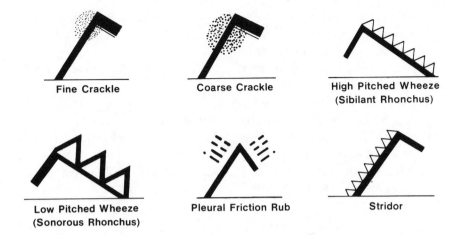

FIGURE 5–27. Diagrammatic summary of common adventitious breath sounds.

To differentiate obstructive from nonobstructive sleep apnea, air flow at the nose and mouth and respiratory effort are assessed. Respiratory effort is gauged with a chest strain gauge, intercostal electromyogram, intraesophageal balloon, and other devices. Air flow is sometimes estimated by recording tracheal breath sounds. If respiratory effort is normal while no air flow is detected, then the apnea is of obstructive origin. If there is no air flow and no muscular activity, then the apnea is nonobstructive (Cummiskey et al., 1982; Kupfer and Reynolds, 1983).

A diagrammatic summary of common adventitious breath sounds is presented in Figure 5–27.

STUDY HELPS

1. What is a crackle? What is the cause of crackling?
2. Name and describe the types of disease associated with (a) early inspiratory crackles and (b) late inspiratory crackles.
3. What is a wheeze? What is the correct mechanism of wheezing?
4. What is the difference between a monophonic wheeze and a polyphonic wheeze?
5. What is stridor? Name and describe the conditions commonly associated with stridor, both in children and in adults.
6. What pathologic condition is associated with a mediastinal crunch?
7. What is the pathologic significance of an inspiratory "squawk"?

8. What is heard in a patient with egophony? What pathologic conditions are associated with egophony? Describe the sound transmutation that produces egophony.

9. Describe whispered pectoriloquy. With what pathologic conditions is it associated?

10. Describe bronchophony and bronchial breathing. With what pathologic conditions are they associated?

11. What effect does emphysema have on the amplitude of breath sounds heard over the chest?

12. What is the significance of crackles heard over the chest after a myocardial infarction, while the patient is still in the coronary care unit?

BIBLIOGRAPHY

Anonymous: Say ninety-nine. *Lancet* [editorial] 2:1258–1259, 1986.

Anonymous: Infectious croup. In *Nelson Textbook of Pediatrics*. 13th ed. Behrman RE, Vaughan VC, Nelson WE (eds). Philadelphia, WB Saunders Company, 1987, pp 887–890.

BERKOW R (ed): *The Merck Manual of Diagnosis and Therapy*. 16th ed. Rahway, NJ, Merck & Company, 1992.

BOHADANA AB, PESLIN R, UFFHOLTZ H: Breath sounds in the clinical assessment of airflow obstruction. *Thorax* 33:345–351, 1978.

CHRISTOPHER KL, WOOD RP, ECKERT RC et al.: Vocal cord dysfunction presenting as asthma. *N Engl J Med* 308:1566–1570, 1983.

CUGELL DW: Sounds of the lungs. *Chest* 73:311–312, 1978.

CUMMISKEY J, WILLIAMS TC, KRUMPE PE et al: The detection and quantification of sleep apnea by tracheal sound recordings. *Am Rev Respir Dis* 126:221–224, 1982.

EARIS JE, MARSH K, PEARSON MG et al.: The inspiratory "squawk" in extrinsic allergic alveolitis and other pulmonary fibroses. *Thorax* 37:923–926, 1982.

EPLER GR, CARRINGTON CB, GAENSLER EA: Crackles (rales) in the interstitial pulmonary diseases. *Chest* 73:333–339, 1978.

FORGACS P: The functional basis of pulmonary sounds. *Chest* 73:399–405, 1978a.

FORGACS P: *Lung Sounds*. London, Baillière Tindall, 1978b.

FRÖSCHELS E, STOCKERT FG: Über ein neues Symptom bei Lungen und Pleurakrankheiten. *Wien Klin Wochenschr* 35:500, 1922.

HUDSON LD, CONN RD, MATSUBARA RS et al.: Rales: Diagnostic uselessness of qualitative adjectives. *Am Rev Respir Dis* 113(2):187, 1976.

JONES FL: Poor breath sounds with good voice sounds. A sign of bronchial stenosis. *Chest* 93(2):312–313, 1988.

KRAMAN SS: The forced expiratory wheeze: Its site of origin and possible association with lung compliance. *Respiration* 44:189–196, 1983.

KRAMAN SS: Lung sounds for the clinician. *Arch Int Med* 146:1411–1412, 1986.

KRUMPE P, FINLEY T, WONG L et al.: The bronchial leak squeak. A new sign for the physical diagnosis of bronchopleurocutaneous fistula. *Chest* 79:336–339, 1981.

KUPFER DJ, REYNOLDS CF: Sleep disorders. *Hosp Pract* 18:101–124, 1983.

LUDMAN H: Hoarseness and stridor. *Br Med J* 282:715–717, 1981.

MARTINI P, MÜLLER H: Studien über das Bronchialatmen. *Dtsch Arch Klin Med* 143:159–173, 1923.

McKUSICK VA, JENKINS JT, WEBB GN: The acoustic basis of the chest examination. Studies by means of sound spectrography. *Am Rev Tuberc* 72:12–34, 1955.

MIKAMI R, MURAO M, CUGELL D, CHRETIEN J, COLE P, MEIER-SYDOW J, MURPHY RLH, LOUDON RG: International symposium on lung sounds. Synopsis of proceedings. *Chest* 92(2):342–345, 1987.

MORI M, KINOSHITA K, MORINARI H et al.: Waveform and spectral analysis of crackles. *Thorax* 35:843–850, 1980.

MUNAKATA M, UKITA H, DOI I, OHTSUKA Y, MASAKI Y, HOMMA Y, KAWAKAMI Y: Spectral and waveform characteristics of fine and coarse crackles. *Thorax* 46(9):651–657, 1991.

MURPHY RL: Auscultation of the lung: Past lessons, future possibilities. *Thorax* 36:99–107, 1981.

NATH AR, CAPEL LH: Inspiratory crackles—early and late. *Thorax* 29:223–227, 1974a.

NATH AR, CAPEL LH: Inspiratory crackles and mechanical events of breathing. *Thorax* 29:695–698, 1974b.

NATH AR, CAPEL LH: Lung crackles in bronchiectasis. *Thorax* 35:694–699, 1980.

PARDEE NE, MARTIN CJ, MORGAN EH: A test of the practical value of estimating breath sound intensity. Breath sounds related to measured ventilatory function. *Chest* 70:341–344, 1976.

PASTERKAMP H, MONTGOMERY M, WIEBICKE W: Nomenclature used by health care professionals to describe breath sounds in asthma. *Chest* 92(2):346–352, 1987.

PASTERKAMP H, WIEBICKE W, FENTON R: Subjective assessment vs. computer analysis of wheezing in asthma. *Chest* 91(3):376–381, 1987.

ROBERTS KB (ed): *Manual of Clinical Problems in Pediatrics*. Boston, Little, Brown & Company, 1979.

ROBERTSON JA, COPE R: Rales, rhonchi, and Laennec. *Lancet* 2:417, 1957.

SHIBLEY GS: New auscultatory sign found in consolidation, or collection of fluid in pulmonary disease. *Chin Med J* 36:1, 1922.

SHIRAI F, KUDOH S, SHIBUYA A et al.: Crackles in asbestos workers: Auscultation and lung sound analysis. *Br J Dis Chest* 75:386–396, 1981.

SPITTER MA, COOK DG, CLARKE SW: Reliability of eliciting physical signs in examination of the chest. *Lancet* 1:873–875, 1988.

THACKER R, KRAMAN SS: The incidence of auscultatory crackles in subjects without lung disease. *Chest* 81:672–674, 1982.

The Multicenter Postinfarction Research Group: Risk stratification and survival after myocardial infarction. *N Engl J Med* 309:331–336, 1983.

WORKUM P, HOLFORD S, DEL BONO E et al.: The prevalence of crackles in young adult females. *Am Rev Respir Dis* 126:921, 1982.

SCRIPT FOR ACCOMPANYING TAPE*

This tape contains recordings of breath sounds that you are likely to hear while examining the chest of both normal individuals and patients with pulmonary disease. To hear the sounds reproduced most realistically, you should listen to the tape through a stethoscope.* Be sure that the earpieces are pointing forward. Then hold the bell 2 to 3 inches from the speaker of your tape recorder. If you place the bell on the speaker, you will hear more noise than breath sounds. If you listen to the sounds without a stethoscope, they will sound unnaturally loud and booming. This phenomenon, known as the Fletcher-Munson effect, is due to the frequency response characteristics of the human ear. On some of the sounds on this tape, you will hear a short beep just before or during **inspiration.**

Listen now to *normal vesicular breath sounds.* . . . Note the relatively soft, low-pitched character of normal vesicular breath sounds, sometimes described as a sighing or gentle rustling. These sounds are heard over most of the peripheral parts of the lung. The inspiratory phase is markedly longer than the expiratory phase. Expiration is much quieter than inspiration, and there is no pause between inspiration and expiration. The term *vesicular* is a misnomer; it arose from experiments performed in the nineteenth century suggesting that these normal sounds originated in the alveoli, then called vesicles. In fact, modern engineering concepts make it more likely that the sounds emanate from the turbulent flow of air in the lobar and segmental bronchi, not the alveoli. Now listen again to normal vesicular breath sounds. . . .

Listen to *bronchial breath sounds.* . . . These characteristically

*Note: While listening to this tape, you may find it helpful to stop the tape recorder, take off your stethoscope, and rest your ears periodically.

130

loud, high-pitched bronchial breath sounds resemble the sound of air blowing through a hollow pipe. Their expiratory phase is louder and longer than their inspiratory phase. They are present normally only over the manubrium, and there is a distinct pause between the inspiratory and expiratory phases. The appearance of bronchial breath sounds over the periphery of the lung may mean abnormal sound transmission because of consolidated lung tissue, as in pneumonia. Now listen to *bronchial breath sounds over the chest of a patient with pneumonia*. Note that the heart sounds are also audible. . . .

These are *bronchovesicular breath sounds*. . . . Bronchovesicular breath sounds are a mixture of bronchial and vesicular sounds. Their inspiratory and expiratory phases are about equal in length. They are normally audible in two places: (1) anteriorly near the mainstem bronchi in the first and second intercostal spaces; and (2) posteriorly between the scapulae. They may be heard elsewhere in the presence of lung consolidation. Listen again to bronchovesicular breath sounds. . . .

The following are *tracheal breath sounds*. . . . Tracheal breath sounds, not usually auscultated, are present over the extrathoracic portion of the trachea. They are very loud, very high-pitched, and have a harsh, hollow quality, the expiratory phase being slightly longer than the inspiratory phase. Listen again to tracheal breath sounds. . . .

Here are *breath sounds over a cavity* in the lung. . . . These sounds are also called amphorous breath sounds. Expiration is equal in length to inspiration but lower in pitch. There is a pause between inspiration and expiration, and the heart tones are audible. Now listen again to amphorous breath sounds. . . .

Crackles are short, explosive, nonmusical sounds. They may be classified as high- or low-pitched. High-pitched crackles are also called fine crackles; low-pitched crackles are also called coarse crackles. Listen now to *high-pitched crackles*. . . . Now listen to *low-pitched crackles*. . . . Crackles are due to the sudden opening of very small airways. Listen again to high-pitched crackles. . . . Listen again to low-pitched crackles. . . .

Crackles may be classified as to position in the respiratory cycle. You will now hear *early inspiratory crackles*. . . . Early inspiratory crackles are characteristic of severe airway obstruction and appear to be produced in the proximal and larger airways. They are not silenced by cough or change of posture. Among the diseases associated with early inspiratory crackles are chronic bronchitis, asthma, and emphysema. Listen again to *early inspiratory crackles*. . . .

The following are *late inspiratory crackles*. . . . Late inspiratory crackles appear to originate in peripheral airways and may occasionally be associated with an end-inspiratory wheeze. Late inspiratory crackles are characteristic of restrictive pulmonary disease and may be heard in interstitial fibrosis, asbestosis, pneumonia, pulmonary congestion of heart failure, pulmonary sarcoidosis, scleroderma, and rheumatoid lung. Listen again to late inspiratory crackles. . . .

Sometimes crackles are produced by the accumulation of secretions in the airway. When the secretions are profuse, the crackles can be heard over the mouth as well as over the chest wall, a sign known to ancient physicians as the *death rattle.* You will now hear a death rattle in a dying patient, over the mouth. . . .

Listen now to the sound of *wheezing.* . . . A wheeze, sometimes called a rhonchus, is a musical pulmonary sound. The musical character is determined by the spectrum of frequencies that make up the sound. The lowest frequency, called the fundamental, sets the pitch of the wheeze. Wheezes may be described as high-pitched, in which case they are also called sibilant rhonchi, or low-pitched, in which case they are also called sonorous rhonchi. Listen to a *high-pitched wheeze.* . . . Now listen to a *low-pitched wheeze.* . . .

Wheezing is produced by a bronchus narrowed to the point of closure, whose opposite walls oscillate between the closed and barely open position. The sound made by a vibrating reed instrument, such as an oboe or the mouthpiece of a child's toy trumpet, is generated in the same manner as a wheeze. If the wheeze is made up of a single musical note, it is called a monophonic wheeze. Listen to the following example of a *monophonic wheeze.* . . . If a wheeze is composed of several dissonant notes starting and ending at the same time, it is called a polyphonic wheeze. All forms of obstructive lung disease may be associated with polyphonic wheezing. Listen to a *polyphonic wheeze.* . . .

Stridor is a particularly loud musical sound of constant pitch. Listen to this example of stridor in a child with croup. . . . Although nothing except its intensity distinguishes stridor from a monophonic wheeze to the ear, stridor comes from obstruction of central airways such as the trachea or larynx. Wheezing is produced in more peripheral airways. Listen again to *stridor.* . . .

Listen to a *pleural friction rub.* . . . The smooth, moist layers of the normal pleura move easily and silently over one another. But when the surface is thickened by fibrin deposits or coarsened by inflammatory or neoplastic cells, the sliding motion is impeded by frictional resistance. The sound produced, the pleural friction rub, resembles the sound of leather sliding on leather. Listen again to a *pleural friction rub.* . . .

The following sound is a *squawk.* . . . Many squawks are inspiratory, but this squawk is both inspiratory and expiratory, louder on inspiration and softer on expiration. The squawk is a musical sound found in some patients with diffuse pulmonary fibrosis, especially if associated with an allergic inflammation of the alveoli known as hypersensitivity pneumonitis. Here is the squawk again. . . .

The presence of a bronchopleurocutaneous fistula may be accompanied by a *bronchial leak squeak,* which you will now hear. . . . The squeak is a high-pitched sound over the affected chest area during a sustained Valsalva maneuver, the pitch being higher in smaller fistulas than in larger fistulas. This squeak was recorded without a stethoscope directly over a fistula. Listen again to a bronchial leak squeak. . . .

Egophony, which is the Greek word for the voice of a goat, refers to the nasal or bleating quality of speech transmitted through consolidated lung tissue, as in pneumonia. Occasionally, egophony will be heard over a pleural effusion where there is collapse of the underlying lung. When egophony occurs, if the patient says E, the letter will sound like A, because there is transmission of the higher frequencies, or formants. First you will hear the letter E spoken over the healthy side. . . . Now you will hear the letter E spoken over the area of consolidation. . . . Now you will hear the sounds as the microphone is moved from one side to the other, starting with the healthy side. . . .

In the normal lung, whispered sounds are not transmitted because they lack the lower frequencies best transmitted by aerated lung tissue, and they are inaudible over the normal chest. However, through airless, consolidated lung tissue the high-pitched whispered sounds above 200 cycles are transmitted, and whispering becomes audible. You will hear this phenomenon, *whispered pectoriloquy*, now. The patient will whisper the words "one, two, three," and you will hear the sound first over the normal lung, . . . then over the consolidated lung. . . . Listen now as we alternate between sides. Note that the heart sounds are clearly audible over the consolidated area.

A few sounds will now be presented as unknowns to test your diagnostic ability. After their presentation, the sounds will be described. You should try to identify each sound before the description is given. Here is the first test sound. . . . Those were normal vesicular breath sounds.

Now here is the second test sound. . . . Those were tracheal breath sounds.

Now here is the third test sound. . . . Those were bronchial breath sounds from the right parasternal area.

Now here is the fourth test sound. . . . That was a wheeze and also some coarse crackles.

Now here is the fifth test sound. . . . Those were fine crackles in a patient with interstitial fibrosis. Note that they persisted well into the last half of inspiration.

Now here is the sixth test sound. . . . That was a pleural friction rub.

ACKNOWLEDGMENTS

1. Normal vesicular breath sounds (courtesy Dr. Roy Donnerberg, Ohio State University, Department of Medicine, Pulmonary Diseases)

2. Bronchial breath sounds, including bronchial breath sounds over the chest of a patient with pneumonia (courtesy Dr. Roy Donnerberg, Ohio State University, Department of Medicine, Pulmonary Diseases; Dr. David W. Cugell, Dr. Earle B. Weiss, and the American College of Chest Physicians)
3. Bronchovesicular breath sounds (courtesy Dr. Roy Donnerberg, Ohio State University, Department of Medicine, Pulmonary Diseases)
4. Tracheal breath sounds (courtesy Dr. Roy Donnerberg, Ohio State University, Department of Medicine, Pulmonary Diseases)
5. Amphorous breath sounds (courtesy Dr. David W. Cugell, Dr. Earle B. Weiss, and the American College of Chest Physicians)
6. High-pitched crackles (courtesy Dr. Roy Donnerberg, Ohio State University, Department of Medicine, Pulmonary Diseases)
7. Low-pitched crackles (courtesy Dr. David W. Cugell, Dr. Earle B. Weiss, and the American College of Chest Physicians)
8. Early inspiratory crackles (courtesy Dr. A. R. Nath)
9. Late inspiratory crackles (courtesy Dr. A. R. Nath)
10. Death rattle (courtesy Dr. Steve S. Kraman)
11. Wheezes (courtesy Dr. David W. Cugell, Dr. Earle B. Weiss, and the American College of Chest Physicians)
12. High-pitched wheeze (courtesy Dr. Roy Donnerberg, Ohio State University, Department of Medicine, Pulmonary Diseases)
13. Low-pitched wheeze (courtesy Dr. Roy Donnerberg, Ohio State University, Department of Medicine, Pulmonary Diseases)
14. Monophonic wheeze
15. Polyphonic wheeze (courtesy Dr. David W. Cugell, Dr. Earle B. Weiss, and the American College of Chest Physicians)
16. Infant stridor (courtesy Dr. David W. Cugell, Dr. Earle B. Weiss, and the American College of Chest Physicians)
17. Pleural friction rub (courtesy Dr. David W. Cugell, Dr. Earle B. Weiss, and the American College of Chest Physicians)
18. Squawk (courtesy Dr. Steve S. Kraman)
19. Bronchial leak squeak (courtesy Dr. Peter Krumpe)
20. Egophony (courtesy Dr. David W. Cugell, Dr. Earle B. Weiss, and the American College of Chest Physicians)
21. Whispered pectoriloquy (courtesy Dr. David W. Cugell, Dr. Earle B. Weiss, and the American College of Chest Physicians)

UNKNOWNS

1. Normal vesicular breath sounds (courtesy Dr. Steve S. Kraman)
2. Tracheal breath sounds (courtesy Dr. Steve S. Kraman)
3. Bronchial breath sounds (courtesy Dr. Steve S. Kraman)
4. Wheeze and coarse crackles (courtesy Dr. Steve S. Kraman)
5. Fine crackles (courtesy Dr. Steve S. Kraman)
6. Pleural friction rub (courtesy Dr. Steve S. Kraman)

GLOSSARY

Achalasia: Failure of the smooth muscle fibers of the gastrointestinal tract to relax at any point of junction of one part with another. An example is the failure of the smooth muscle fibers of the lower esophagus to relax, called *achalasia of the esophagus*, which is characterized by dilatation and hypertrophy of the esophagus above an atrophic lower segment (megaesophagus).

Adduction: A drawing together.

Aneurysm: A sac formed by the dilatation of the walls of an artery or of a vein filled with blood. A dissecting aneurysm is one in which the blood is forced between the coats of an artery.

Angina pectoris: A paroxysmal thoracic pain, with a feeling of suffocation and impending death. This is usually due to insufficient oxygen reaching the heart muscle and is precipitated by effort or excitement.

Antigen: A high molecular weight substance or complex, usually protein or protein polysaccharide in nature. When it is foreign to the blood stream of an animal, on gaining access to the tissues of such an animal it stimulates the formation of specific antibody and reacts specifically in vivo or in vitro with its homologous antibody.

Aorta: The main trunk from which the systemic arterial system proceeds. It arises from the left ventricle of the heart, passes upward, bends over, and passes down through the thorax and abdomen to the fourth lumbar vertebra, where it divides into the two common iliac arteries.

Apex (pulmonary): The rounded upper extremity of either lung, extending upward as high as the first thoracic vertebra; also called *lung apex.*

Apnea: The transient cessation of breathing.

Arytenoids: A pair of ladle-shaped cartilages that form part of the larynx.

Asbestos: A fibrous magnesium and calcium silicate often used for thermal insulation.

Ascites: Effusion of serous fluid into the abdominal cavity.

Atelectasis: Incomplete expansion or collapse of the lung.

Atrophy: A defect or failure of nutrition manifested as a wasting away or diminution in the size of a cell, tissue, organ, or part.

Axilla: The small hollow beneath the arm, where it joins the body at the shoulder; also called *armpit.*

Binaural: Pertaining to both ears.

Biopsy: The removal and examination, usually microscopic, of tissue or other material from the living body for purposes of diagnosis.

Bronchiectasis: A chronic dilatation of the bronchi or bronchioles.

Bronchiole: One of the finer subdivisions of the branched bronchial tree.

Bronchitis: An inflammation of the bronchial tubes.

Bronchophony: The sound of the voice as heard through the stethoscope applied over a healthy bronchus. When heard elsewhere, it indicates solidification of the lung tissue.

Bronchopleural: Pertaining to a bronchus and the pleura, or communicating with a bronchus and the pleural cavity, as a bronchopleural fistula.

Bronchus: One of the larger air passages within the lungs.

Bulla: In the lung, a bubble-shaped abnormality often associated with emphysema.

Carina: A keel-shaped structure, a projection of the lowest tracheal cartilage, which forms a prominent semilunar ridge running anteroposteriorly between the orifices of the two bronchi.

Cochlea: The essential organ of hearing, a spiral-wound tube that resembles a snail shell and forms part of the inner ear.

Consolidation: Solidification, as of a lung in pneumonia.

Costochondral: Pertaining to a rib and its cartilage.

Crackle: A short, explosive, nonmusical sound heard over the chest, and sometimes at the mouth.

Crepitation: A crackling noise, as would be made when there is air in subcutaneous tissue or when the ends of fractured bones rub together.

Cyanosis: A bluish discoloration of skin and mucous membranes due to excessive concentration of reduced hemoglobin in the blood.

Diaphragm: The musculomembranous partition separating the abdominal and thoracic cavities.

Diastole: The dilatation, or period of dilatation, of the heart, especially that of the ventricles. It coincides with the interval between the second and first heart sounds.

Dyspnea: Difficult or labored breathing.

Edema: Swelling.

Effusion: The escape of fluid into a part or tissue.

Egophony: A bleating quality of voice observed in auscultation in certain cases of lung consolidation.

Embolus: A clot or other plug carried by the blood from another vessel and forced into a smaller one so as to obstruct the circulation.

Emphysema: A swelling or inflation due to the presence of air. This applies especially to a pathologic condition of the lungs, pulmonary emphysema, in which there is an increase beyond normal in the size of air spaces distal to the terminal bronchioles, either from dilatation of the alveoli or from destruction of their walls.

Empyema: Accumulation of pus in a cavity of the body, especially in the chest (pyothorax).

Encephalitis: Inflammation of the brain.

Epiglottis: An elastic cartilage, covered by mucous membrane, that forms the upper part of the larynx and guards the glottis during swallowing.

Esophagus: The musculomembranous passage extending from the pharynx to the stomach.

Etiology: cause.

Fibrosis: The formation of fibrous tissue.

Fistula: An abnormal passage or

communication, usually between two internal organs, or leading from an internal organ to the surface of the body. It is frequently designated according to the organs or parts with which it communicates, for example, bronchocutaneous.

Fremitus: A thrill or vibration, especially one that is perceptible on palpation.

Glottis: The vocal apparatus of the larynx, consisting of the true vocal cords (vocal folds) and the opening between them (rima glottidis).

Goiter: An enlargement of the thyroid gland, causing a swelling in the front part of the neck.

Granuloma: A localized nodule of inflammatory tissue showing the process of granulation. A caseating granuloma is associated with tuberculosis; a noncaseating granuloma is seen in sarcoidosis.

Hematemesis: The vomiting of blood.

Hemoptysis: The coughing up of blood or blood-stained sputum.

Hemothorax: Blood in the pleural space.

Hiatus hernia: Protrusion of any structure through the esophageal hiatus of the diaphragm.

Hilum: A recess in the lung just above the cardiac impression.

Hypertrophy: The morbid enlargement or overgrowth of an organ or part due to an increase in size of its constituent cells.

Idiopathic: Of unknown cause.

Intensity: An objective assessment determined by the amplitude of the vibrations, their generating source, the distance traveled, and the medium through which they travel.

Intercostal: Situated between the ribs.

Intubation: The insertion of a tube into the airway to facilitate breathing.

Kyphosis: A condition characterized by an abnormally increased convexity in the curvature of the thoracic spine as viewed from the side; also called a *humpback*.

Larynx: The musculocartilaginous structure, lined with mucous membrane, situated at the top of the trachea and below the root of the tongue and the hyoid bone. It is the essential sphincter guarding the entrance into the trachea and functions secondarily as the organ of the voice.

Mediastinum: The mass of tissues and organs separating the two lungs between the sternum in front and the vertebral column behind and from the thoracic inlet above to the diaphragm below. It contains the heart and its large vessels, as well as the trachea, esophagus, thymus, lymph nodes, and other structures and tissues. It is divided into anterior, middle, posterior, and superior regions.

Meningitis: An inflammation of the meninges, the three membranes (dura mater, pia mater, and arachnoid) that envelop the brain and the spinal cord.

Mesothelioma: A primary tumor of the cells forming the lining of the peritoneum, pericardium, or pleura.

Mitral stenosis: Narrowing of the left atrioventricular orifice.

Mycoplasma: A taxonomic name given a genus including the pleuropneumonia-like organisms (PPLO) and separated into 15 species on the basis of source, glucose fermentation, and growth on agar media.

Myocardial infarction: An area of coagulation necrosis in the heart muscle due to an interruption of the blood supply to that area.

Nasopharynx: That part of the pharynx above the level of the soft palate, communicating with the posterior nares and the auditory tube.

Neoplastic: Pertaining to a new and abnormal growth, such as a tumor.

Neuritis: Inflammation of a nerve.

Noncaseating: A degenerative change not having the consistency of cheese.

Oncotic: Pertaining to, caused by, or marked by swelling.

Orthopnea: The need to sit up in order to avoid breathing difficulty; associated with heart disease.

Paroxysm: A sudden recurrence or intensification of symptoms.

Pectoriloquy: Transmission of the sound of spoken words through the chest wall. Whispered pectoriloquy is the transmission of the sound of whispered words through the chest wall and indicates lung consolidation.

Pericardium: The fibroserous sac that surrounds the heart, comprising an external layer of dense fibrous tissue (fibrous pericardium) and an inner serous layer (serous pericardium). The visceral pericardium is the inner layer of the serous pericardium in contact with the heart. The parietal pericardium is that layer in contact with the fibrous pericardium.

Peritoneum: The serous membrane lining the abdominopelvic walls and investing the viscera.

pH: The symbol commonly used in expressing hydrogen ion concentration, the measure of alkalinity and acidity. It signifies the logarithm of the reciprocal of the hydrogen ion concentration in gram molecules per liter of solution. pH 7 is the neutral point; above 7, alkalinity increases; below 7, acidity increases.

Pharynx: The musculomembranous sac between the mouth and nares and the esophagus. It is continuous below with the esophagus, and above it communicates with the larynx, mouth, nasal passages, and auditory tubes.

Pleura: The serous membrane investing the lungs and lining the thoracic cavity, completely enclosing a potential space known as the pleural cavity. The parietal pleura is that portion lining the walls of the thoracic cavity. The visceral pleura is that portion investing the lungs and lining their fissures, completely separating the different lobes.

Pneumothorax: An accumulation of air in the pleural cavity, which may occur spontaneously or as a result of trauma, a pathologic process, or deliberate induction.

Precordium: The region over the heart or stomach; the epigastrium and lower part of the thorax.

Prodrome: A premonitory symptom or precursor; a symptom indicating the onset of a disease.

Psittacosis: A microbial disease first observed in parrots and known to be communicated by them to man and later discovered to exist in other birds and domestic fowl.

Purulent: Consisting of or containing pus.

Resonance: The prolongation and intensification of sound produced by the transmission of its vibrations to a cavity.

Rhonchus: A musical pulmonary sound (also called a wheeze).

Scoliosis: An appreciable lateral deviation in the normally straight vertical line of the spine.

Sibilant: High-pitched.

Sonorous: Low-pitched.

Sphincter: A ringlike band of muscle fibers that constricts a passage or closes a natural orifice.

Sputum: Matter ejected from the lungs, bronchi, and trachea through the mouth.

Stenosis: A narrowing.

Sternum: A longitudinal unpaired plate of bone forming the middle of the anterior wall of the thorax. It articulates above with the clavicles and along the sides with the cartilages of the first seven ribs and consists of three portions— the manubrium, the body, and the xiphoid process.

Syncope: A sudden loss of strength; a temporary suspension of consciousness due to cerebral anemia; a faint.

Systole: The contraction, or period of contraction, of the heart, especially that of the ventricles. It corresponds with the interval between the first and second heart sounds, during which the blood is forced into the aorta and pulmonary trunk.

Thorax: The part of the body between the neck and the respiratory diaphragm, encased by the ribs; the chest.

Thyroidectomy: Removal of part or all of the thyroid gland.

Tomography: A special x-ray technique to show detail in images of structures lying in a predetermined plane of tissue, while blurring or eliminating detail in images of stuctures in other planes. It is also called *body section roentgenography*.

Trachea: The cartilaginous and membranous tube descending from the larynx to the bronchi.

Tracheostomy: Surgical creation of an opening into the trachea through the neck for insertion of a tube to facilitate the passage of air into the lungs or for the evacuation of secretions.

Unilateral: One-sided.

Valsalva maneuver: Expiratory effort against a closed glottis.

Varices (plural of varix): Enlarged and tortuous vessels. Esophageal varices are enlarged and tortuous veins.

Viscosity: A physical property of a substance that is dependent on the friction of its component molecules as they slide by one another. For example, cold maple syrup is more viscous than warm water.

Wheeze: A musical pulmonary sound (also called a rhonchus).

INDEX

Page numbers in italics refer to illustrations.
Page numbers followed by t refer to tables.